THE EXPERTS PRAISE

CONFRONTING MITRAL VALVE PROLAPSE SYNDROME

❐

"A blessing to my practice. . . . We order this text by the case for our patients. They are delighted that someone has an obvious understanding of a problem that has frustrated many of them for years. . . . I can strongly recommend this text to patients with MVP/dysautonomia and to physicians who treat them."
—Gary S. Niess, M.D., F.A.C.C.,
Mecklenburg Cardiovascular
Consultants, Director Coronary Care Unit,
Belk Heart Center,
Presbyterian Hospital, Charlotte, North Carolina

❐

"Lyn Frederickson's book contains a wealth of information about mitral valve prolapse; it is a great help to both patients who have this condition and the physicians who treat them."
—Michael Colandrea, M.D., cardiologist,
Good Samaritan Hospital, Chicago

CONFRONTING
MITRAL VALVE
PROLAPSE
SYNDROME

Lyn Frederickson, M.S.N.

WARNER BOOKS

A Time Warner Company

The advice in this book can be a valuable addition to your doctor's advice, and is designed for your use under his or her care and direction.

It is with deep respect and affection that I dedicate this work to my teacher and friend H. Cecil Coghlan, M.D., Professor of Medicine/Cardiology-University of Alabama in Birmingham.

Dr. Coghlan taught me everything about mitral valve prolapse syndrome as well as valuable lessons in courage and humility. Dr. Coghlan recognized that MVP was a very real problem far before anyone else and had the professional courage and integrity to pursue answers about this problem even when it was not popular to do so.

The world truly is a better place because of Dr. Coghlan.
I feel very honored to have worked with him.

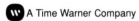

Warner Books Edition

This Warner Books edition is published by arrangement with Slawson Communications, Inc., 165 Vallecitos de Oro, San Marcos, CA 92069

Warner Books, Inc., 1271 Avenue of the Americas, New York, NY 10020

Ⓦ A Time Warner Company

Printed in the United States of America

First Warner Books Printing: August 1992

10 9 8 7 6 5

Library of Congress Cataloging in Publication Data
Frederickson, Lyn.
    Confronting mitral valve prolapse syndrome / Lyn Frederickson. --
Warner Books ed.
        p.   cm.
    Originally published : Confronting mitral valve prolapse. San
Marcos, CA : Avant Books, c1988.
    Includes bibliographical references and index.
    ISBN 0-446-39407-6
    1. Mitral valve--Displacement--Popular works.   I. Title.
RC685.V2F37   1992
616.1 ' 25--dc20   92-9871
                                                                CIP

Cover design by Julia Kushnirsky
Cover photograph by Stock Market

Contents

Acknowledgments

It would be impossible to complete such a project as this book without help. I have had the privilege of working with a number of really outstanding physicians through the years and would like to share the credit for this project with a few of them. Dr. H. Cecil Coghlan has been a friend and colleague for a number of years and really stimulated my interest in mitral valve prolapse patients. I sincerely respect and admire his compassion and his inquiring mind in dealing with this problem. Dr. Richard O. Russell has been a source of continuing of support throughout this project, and I will always think of him as the "physician's-physician" and the quintessential gentleman. Dr. Phillip C. Watkins shared my vision for a Mitral Valve Prolapse Center and had the energy and persuasive ability to get the job done.

Many thanks to the Baptist Medical Centers of Alabama for their commitment to public service. They supported me in my efforts to establish the Mitral Valve Prolapse Center. The staff of the Center deserve my most sincere thanks for lending their smiling faces for the photographs in this book as well as for their willingness to pick up the slack when I have had to be away. A very special thanks to those that assisted with the preparation of this manuscript. It is rare that an individual is fortunate enough to get up in the morning and really look forward to going to work. I am indeed blessed to feel that way, and to a large degree the staff of the Center is responsible for this attitude. Thanks to Rita Yerby for the art work and to Jerry Goldstein for the photographs.

Last, but not least, a sincere thanks to my best friend and husband Dr. Bob Frederickson, for his support and encouragement and for tolerating take-out Chinese food night after night so that I could work. A special thanks also for taking me to the mountains to save my sanity. No woman could ask for a better partner for life. And to my children, Mark and Amy—I love you both.

Lyn Frederickson

Foreword

Confronting Mitral Valve Prolapse: Mysterious Heart Condition of the Young and Healthy by Lyn Frederickson helps to clarify the alarming symptoms of this common medical syndrome better than any treatise I know. It is written for the patient and for her or his family in readable, understandable language, yet underlying it is a depth of professional perception of this syndrome accumulated by well over a decade of talking with and counseling patients having these symptoms. Mrs. Frederickson's expertise and understanding spring from insight gained in a university setting working with Dr. Cecil Coghlan, Professor of Medicine at the University of Alabama in Birmingham, and in a large private referral clinic. Her solid background in cardiovascular nursing and her personal warmth are both apparent in this unique volume.

Mrs. Frederickson was among the first persons anywhere to sense the wider implications of the varied and frightening feelings of individuals with the mitral valve prolapse syndrome, or dysautonomia. She recognized that the sensations of chest pain, palpitation, dizziness, numbness in an arm or fingers, feelings of unreality, alternating constipation and diarrhea, occasional sleep disturbances, extreme anxiety and panic attacks were manifestations of a disturbance, imbalance, or hypersensitivity of the involuntary nervous system — the autonomic nervous system. Hence the name dysautonomia.

It is clear that a broad approach to helping patients improve begins with increasing the level of their own understanding and recognition of their feelings. Additionally, five avenues of therapy, faithfully pursued, help patients improve. These five are (a) maintenance of an increased level of fitness or stamina by a program of isotonic exercise, (b) total avoidance of caffeine, (c) maintenance of a high fluid intake, up to eight glasses of fluid a day, (d) avoidance of sweets, combined with appropriate nutritional intake with three meals a day and small between meal snacks, and (e) medication, if necessary, to help alleviate some of the disconcerting sensations. Mrs. Frederickson eloquently explores each of these avenues and explains the role of each.

Chronic stress and an individual's response to it, both conscious and unconscious, seem to underlie and often to trigger these frightening feelings associated with mitral valve prolapse syndrome. A vitally important factor in dealing with this syndrome is an increased understanding or realization of what is going on in one's body in response to the environment, both external and internal. This book accomplishes just that.

> Richard O. Russell Jr., M.D.
> Clinical Professor of Medicine
> University of Alabama at Birmingham

❑ ❑ ❑

Mitral Valve Prolapse is probably the most common inherited cardiovascular problem in the United States today. It is without a doubt one of the most poorly understood conditions affecting the population as well. The typical patient with mitral valve prolapse syndrome sees multiple physicians with her problems and in all too many cases is told that she has nothing to worry about or, even worse, that this is "all in your head."

It is very important for the patient who has this condition to understand that this is the result of the body's failure to perform its normal regulating processes. By understanding this and realizing that there are things that can be done to correct this, the patient can resume a normal lifestyle. In all too many cases the patient is misdiagnosed or treated incompletely. This book by Lyn Frederickson will help you to understand how mitral valve prolapse syndrome can affect you in so many different ways. More importantly it will show you some lifestyle changes that can cause some meaningful improvements in your condition.

One of the most important parts in treating the patient with mitral valve prolapse syndrome is education. In many cases the medical community has been slow to recognize how devastating the symptoms can be to some patients. However, by learning to recognize what is going on within your body and more importantly what to do about it you can take steps to begin to improve on your own.

> Phillip C. Watkins, M.D.
> Cardiologist
> Medical Director-Mitral Valve Prolapse Center

Introduction

Several years ago I was hired by a large University Medical Center to establish and manage a laboratory specializing in the testing and treatment of patients with the condition known as mitral valve prolapse (MVP). I knew little about this condition even though I had previously been a cardiovascular nurse specialist. But I did know, for example, that these patients were usually young, female, and disliked as patients by the medical staff. From the relatively few medical articles available about MVP I learned that this was a very common variation in the shape of the mitral valve of the heart and was of almost no consequence to the patient's longevity. According to most studies, in fact, it is the most common cardiac variation, occurring in at least 10 percent of the entire population. I was asked to see these patients for counseling and reassurance and to enroll them in a special exercise program, along with my cardiac patients.

Although the patients with MVP benefitted greatly from exercise, it was difficult to conduct an exercise program for these patients at the same time as one for 50- to 70-year old patients with other cardiac problems. The cardiac patients were always in better shape and could "exercise circles" around a patient with prolapse. In fact, the MVP patients had numerous vague symptoms, such as fatigue and chest pains, that were difficult to understand. Initially, my job was to reassure the patients as to the harmless nature of their condition and to "whip them back into shape."

Then, along came Jane (a pseudonym). Jane certainly changed my attitude toward patients with MVP and most probably my career as well. She was an attractive redhead in her fifties with a twinkle in her eye and a lovely smile. For Jane and me it was friendship at first sight, rather than the traditional patient-therapist relationship. The word "charm" could have been invented to describe Jane. She was highly intelligent and loved life. She was deeply involved in her community and her grown children. Her loving husband was totally supportive of her. Jane didn't flow through life, she attacked it. She was very active in her local crisis intervention center and played bridge like an assassin. She also had one of the worst cases of mitral valve prolapse syndrome (fatigue, chest pains, and so forth) that I had ever seen. It was clear immediately that her case was not reflective of a neurotic person who needed an excuse to avoid life, but instead indicated a real problem that could have a devastating impact on her lifestyle. It was also clear that it was uniformly misunderstood by everyone around her. Jane opened my mind to the problem of the prolapse patient.

I began not just *talking* to my patients, but also *listening* to what they had to say. I read everything I could get my hands on about the problem (there was almost nothing) and studied the diagnostic tests I was performing to pick up patterns and clearly define the problem. Slowly I began to recognize a pattern in the symptoms of these patients. There was indeed a difference between the MVP patient and other people. The reason for this was not clear to me. Many had been labeled neurotics and "doctor shoppers," implying that they went from one physician to another looking for answers they wanted to hear, or worse yet, medications to cure them. Many had a rough time maintaining marriages or jobs because of fatigue and other frightening symptoms. Most had been on numerous medications, and many, if not most, had been advised that they should seek psychiatric help. Patients were generally frightened and usually passive. They were embarrassed to tell of their strange symptoms, or the fact that they were not improving on the medications that had been prescribed for them. But, given a sympathetic ear, they would pour forth from one to two hours of information about their experiences and symptoms. Every patient, without exception, pleaded for something written about the problem that they could take home and share with their family and friends. They were anxious to know what they could do to help solve the problem. There was, of course, no such material available.

I continued my work with these patients for several years before deciding to write this book. When I left the university to establish the first Mitral Valve Prolapse Center, I began to compile my experiences. I have addressed the book primarily to people with MVP. The "you" I speak to is the person who has MVP and who may be living with some or all of the symptoms described. However, the book can also be very helpful to family, friends, and care-givers of MVP patients.

The book is organized as follows:

- Chapters 1 and 2 define MVP and the dysautonomia associated with it, and describe their impact on patients' lives.

- Chapter 3 provides suggestions for choosing a physician and establishing and maintaining a good relationship with him or her. This chapter also provides clues to help you know when it's appropriate to seek a second opinion or change doctors.

- Chapters 4, 5, 6, and 7 describe the roles of exercise, diet, medication, and positive mental attitude in controlling MVP symptoms. Of these four components of treatment, medication may sometimes be omitted. The other three are so closely interrelated that it is difficult or impossible to separate them and identify one that is most important. All are vital. Chapter 4 suggests specific exercises for the MVP patient and provides an exercise record form for you to use. Chapter 5 provides useful menus and recipes as well as dietary record forms to help track and improve food habits.

- Chapter 8 discusses anxiety and panic attacks — what they are and how they are treated. Panic attack can be psychologically and socially debilitating, and may require special treatment beyond that covered in Chapters 4 through 7.

- Chapter 9 sums up the approach to treatment of MVP symptoms.

- Chapter 10 provides answers to twenty of the questions asked most often about MVP.

- The "Glossary" defines some of the more specialized terms used in the book. Although these terms are defined in the text as they are introduced, the "Glossary" can be helpful if you need help recalling the exact meaning of a word.

- The "Suggested Reading" list includes sources of further information on many of the topics covered in this book. Use it to find books about the specific subjects that interest you most.

The goal of this book is to provide a comprehensive approach for patients with MVP to deal with this problem, to give you all the information you need to regain control of your life and to maximize your potential. This you can do! (Hundreds of patients have shared their experiences with me, enabling this book to become a reality, and it is to these patients that this book is dedicated.)

1 What Is Mitral Valve Prolapse?

In a little more than 10 percent of the population, there is a slight variation in the shape or structure of the mitral valve of the heart (Figure 1-1).

This condition is known as *mitral valve prolapse* (*MVP*). It is said to be the most common cardiac variation. In people without MVP, when the lower part of the heart contracts, the mitral valve remains firm and allows no blood to leak back into the upper chambers. When there is MVP, there is a slight variation in shape of the mitral valve that allows one part of the valve, a leaflet, to billow somewhat back into the upper chamber during contraction of the ventricle. This protrusion can often be heard through the physician's stethoscope, and the sound is known as a "click." There may also be a slight, usually insignificant leak of the valve during contraction of the ventricle, which may also be heard by a stethoscope as a soft murmur. This structural variation has many other names including *floppy valve syndrome*, *click-murmur syndrome*, and *Barlow's syndrome*. I do not refer to this condition as a disease, because it is so common and generally of no consequence. The variation in the shape of the mitral valve is a condition that is hereditary and may appear in various members of a family. Whether someone with MVP has

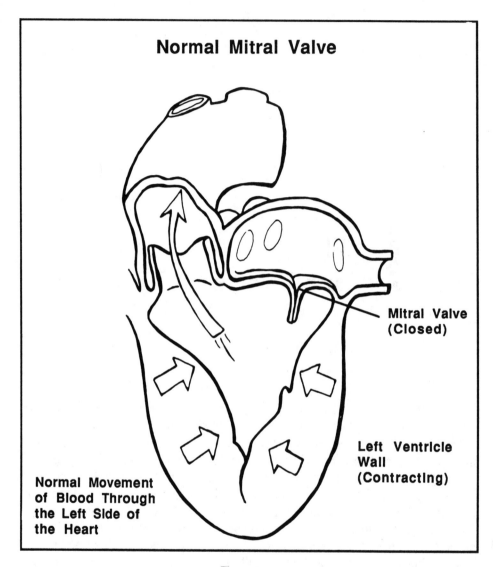

Normal Mitral Valve

Mitral Valve
(Closed)

Left Ventricle
Wall
(Contracting)

Normal Movement
of Blood Through
the Left Side of
the Heart

Figure 1-1a

symptoms or not is thought to be due to a number of environmental variables that will be discussed in detail later. MVP is **not life threatening**, it is a very common condition, and it is usually not even recognized. It may, however, be *lifestyle threatening*.

There is a continuum for MVP.

On one end of the continuum are the vast numbers of people with the mitral

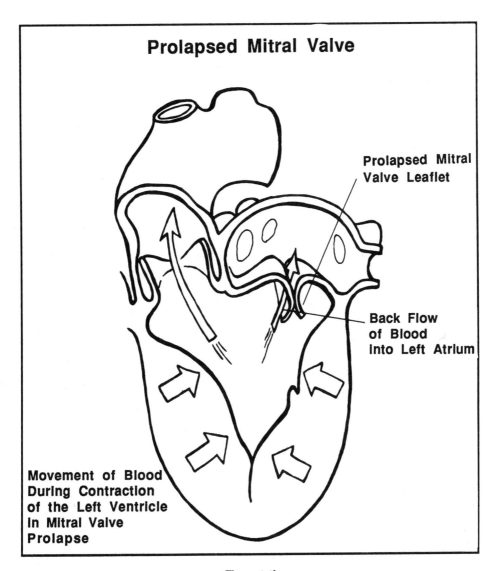

Prolapsed Mitral Valve

Prolapsed Mitral
Valve Leaflet

Back Flow
of Blood
Into Left Atrium

Movement of Blood
During Contraction
of the Left Ventricle
In Mitral Valve
Prolapse

Figure 1-1b

valve structural variation and never any hint of symptoms. On the other end of the continuum, are very small numbers of people who have more severe structural problems that may progress to the point that surgical replacement of the heart valve is required. This is an **extremely small number**. I would also place at this end of the continuum those patients who have very severe symptoms such as irregularity of the heart rate that requires therapy. Once again, these cases are not very common.

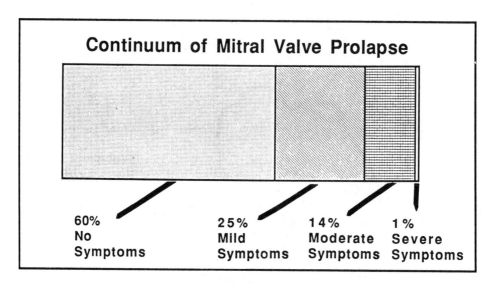

Figure 1-2

In the center of the continuum lie the vast majority of MVP patients. These people may have occasional symptoms that are mildly to moderately uncomfortable. I must emphasize once again that this is not a **life-threatening** condition. But the symptoms can be so frightening or uncomfortable that they interfere with the patient's ability to enjoy a normal life. As you will learn as you read on, this need never be so.

About the Heart

Before one can understand MVP, one needs to look first at the basic structure and function of the heart. It was not until 1628 when William Harvey published his book describing the circulation of the blood and the workings of the heart that people knew what the heart did or how it worked. Until that time people considered the heart to be a place in the body where love and courage were felt, perhaps because it is in the breast that one feels the pangs of passion or unrequited love or surges of valor. Until Harvey's discovery, no one recognized the heart to be one of the most powerful parts of the body. Even today the heart is viewed with awe and great mystery. The average person considers any condition that even remotely involves the heart to be life threatening.

The heart is a pump not much larger than a clenched fist, weighing approximately one-half pound. Its job is to pump blood continuously and steadily to all parts of the body for tissue nourishment and removal of waste products. The heart is located in the front of the chest under the breastbone, and lies more to the left than to the right side. It is protected by the bony structure of the rib cage. The tough muscular wall of the heart is called the *myocardium*(Figure 1-3). Lining the myocardium is a thin strong membrane, the *endocardium*. The myocardium is surrounded by a tough fibrous bag, the *pericardium*.

The pericardium is filled with a small amount of fluid that cushions and supports the heart as it beats. The heart is a hollow organ. A solid partition of muscle, the *septum*, divides the heart cavity into the right heart and left heart chambers. The shaded area in Figure 1-4 represents the right heart, while the non-shaded area represents the left heart. Each side of the heart can be thought of as a separate pump consisting of two hollow chambers, one above the other. The lower chamber on each side is the *ventricle*, the main pumping chamber, while the upper chamber on each side is the *atrium*, or collecting chamber. The upper and lower chambers of the heart are separated by valves that allows the blood to flow in only one direction. The valve on the right side of the heart is the *tricuspid valve*, and the valve on the left side of the heart is the *mitral valve*. The right side of the heart receives blood from all over the body and pumps it to the lungs to discharge carbon dioxide and pick up oxygen. The newly oxygenated blood then returns to the left side of the heart and is pumped to all parts of the body.

By following the arrows in Figure 1-4, you can see that the blood returning from the body to the heart enters the right atrium through the great veins, the *venae cavae* (plural of vena cava).

The blood flows into the upper chamber and down through the tricuspid valve into the right ventricle. The blood is forced into the lungs by the contraction of the right ventricle. After the blood is replenished with oxygen in the lungs, it returns to the heart through the pulmonary veins into the upper chamber. It flows down through the mitral valve into the left ventricle. The mitral valve then closes and, with left ventricular contraction, blood is forced out the aorta to all parts of the body.

About the Nervous System

It is important to understand a few things about the nervous system and the way it is related to the heart and circulation in order to understand the symptoms of MVP. The nervous system has two major components, the *voluntary nervous system* and the *involuntary nervous system*. Many of the differences are obvious from the names of the two systems. The voluntary nervous system controls all actions and activities under voluntary control, such as nerve messages from the brain to the muscle and back again that enable us to stand, walk, and talk. The nervous system

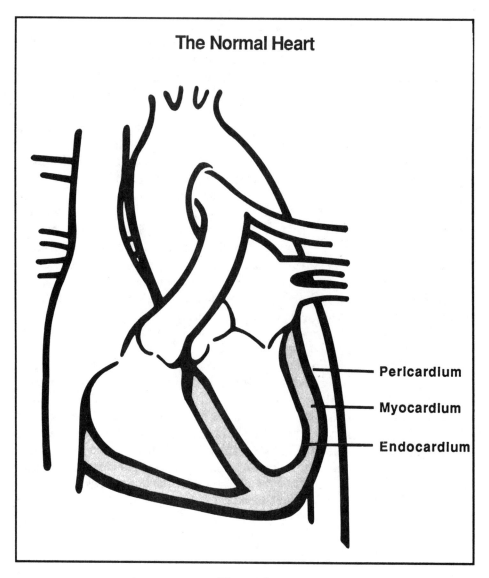

The Normal Heart

Pericardium

Myocardium

Endocardium

Figure 1-3

is extremely complex. It sends tiny impulses that travel very rapidly from the nerve endings in your finger tip (for example), to the brain, telling the brain that the tip of the finger is on a very hot stove. The brain quickly sends the signal telling your arm to contract and pull your finger away from the stove. Other signals make you

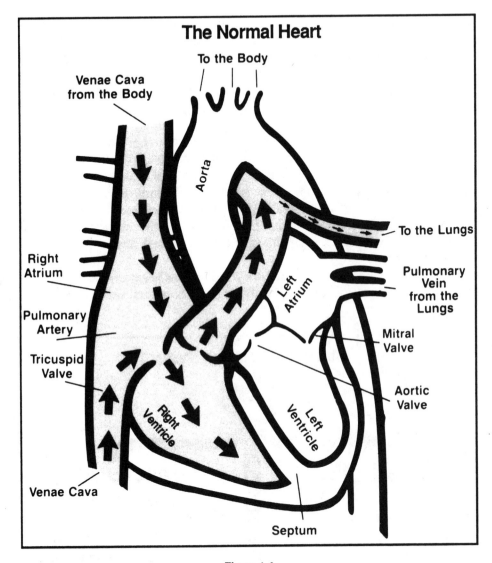

The Normal Heart

To the Body

Venae Cava from the Body

Aorta

To the Lungs

Right Atrium

Pulmonary Vein from the Lungs

Left Atrium

Pulmonary Artery

Mitral Valve

Tricuspid Valve

Aortic Valve

Right Ventricle

Left Ventricle

Venae Cava

Septum

Figure 1-4

move your finger to your mouth to cool the burn. The nervous system is like a great computer far more sophisticated than anything devised by man.

The involuntary nervous system, also known as the *autonomic nervous system*, is perhaps even more complex, controlling most bodily functions not generally considered to be under conscious control. Its functions include regulation of sweating, blood vessel contraction and relaxation, heart rate, dilation and contraction of the pupil of the eye, sleep-wakefulness balance, and many others. Here is an example of autonomic nervous system function: The normal person gets out of bed in the morning, and after a full night's rest, his or her heart rate accelerates 5 to 10 percent and the blood vessels in the arms and legs constrict slightly to maintain the blood pressure upon standing. This autonomic nervous system function prevents fainting every time one stands.

In reality, all systems of the body are under the control of the autonomic nervous system to some degree. There are two major components of the involuntary, or autonomic, nervous system. To simplify, these can be thought of as the accelerator and the brake of the system. The accelerator, or the *sympathetic nervous system*, speeds up the system; the brake, or the *parasympathetic nervous system*, slows the system (Figure 1-5). Neither component is ever in complete control; the two are constantly balancing each other to a greater or lesser degree, depending on the circumstances.

For example, imagine that one of our ancestors was being attacked by a saber-toothed tiger. The accelerator, or sympathetic nervous system, would be activated

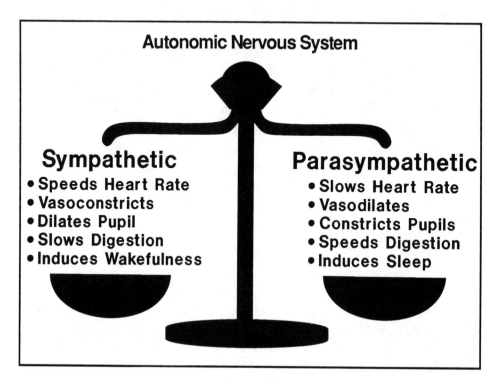

Figure 1-5

and would pour great amounts of adrenalin into the blood. The adrenalin and other nerve signals would increase the heart rate for better blood supply to the muscles, dilate the pupils for better vision, and shut down blood supply to the intestines — after all, first things first!

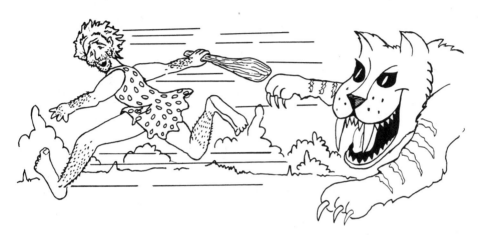

These changes would allow our ancestor to run fast, see well, and, with a little luck, escape the tiger. When he returned to his cave and relaxed, the braking part or the parasympathetic nervous system would be activated. His blood would be flooded with *acetylcholine*, a chemical that would slow the heart rate down to the appropriate level, return the blood supply to the intestines and the other internal organs, and bring the system back down to a baseline level.

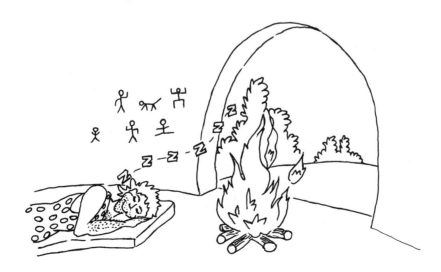

Dysautonomia

In reality, neither the sympathetic nor the parasympathetic nervous system is ever in complete control. Rather, they complement each other to meet the ever-changing needs of an individual's body. The autonomic nervous system serves as the fine-tuning mechanism of the body. A slight problem in this system can lead to an imbalance known as *dysautonomia* (Figure 1-6).

At the same time that the mitral valve of the heart is formed in the unborn baby, the autonomic nervous system is also being formed. Frequently, when there is a slight variation in structure of the heart valve, there is also a slight variation in the function or balance of the autonomic nervous system. Once again, this imbalance is not life threatening, but it can result in a number of symptoms that are commonly associated with MVP.

In fact, almost all of the symptoms of mitral valve prolapse syndrome are due to a slight imbalance of the autonomic nervous system. This imbalance is called *dysautonomia*.

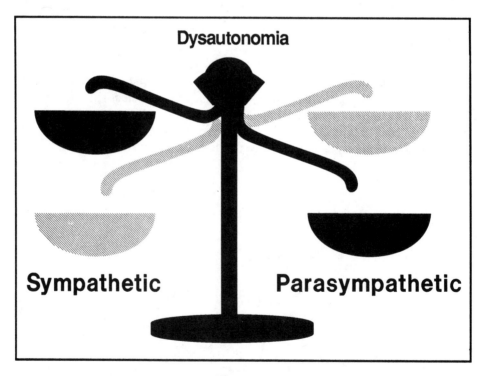

Figure 1-6

The autonomic nervous system is extremely complex. It maintains a delicate balance in response to factors such as stress level, nutritional status, and hormonal balance of the body. As one can easily imagine, there are a number of ways the two components (sympathetic and the parasympathetic) of this delicate system could be out of balance, resulting in dysautonomia. The sympathetic, or accelerator system, could be too active, and the parasympathetic, or brake system, could be not active enough, resulting in inappropriate response of the nervous system. Or both systems could be too active or underactive. In patients with dysautonomia, there is usually a predominant pattern in this imbalance that can be identified and can enable the physician to select a medication that is appropriate for the specific type of dysautonomia. The pattern of dysautonomia may change over time, and the degree to which there is an imbalance may also change over time. The only reliable way to determine the pattern type and the severity is by autonomic nervous system testing, which will be described in detail later in the book.

There are many causes of dysautonomia, but two in particular should be mentioned here. Neither is in any way the result of mitral valve prolapse. Diabetes and coronary heart disease both damage the tiny nerves and therefore result in inappropriate responses of the autonomic nervous system. This kind of dysautonomia is not the same as MVP dysautonomia, either in cause or in consequences.

A History of MVP Syndrome

MVP is seen in all age groups, but most commonly in young adult females. This condition has been around for a long time. Historical novels refer to females who were prone to "the vapors" or "swooning." A similar condition was described during the Civil War when young male soldiers were subjected to the hardships of war and stress. They complained of profound fatigue, shortness of breath, chest pain, and fluttery heartbeats. The term *soldier's heart* was used to describe this condition. During and after World War I in England, hospitals were established to handle the large numbers of young soldiers who were returning from the war with this condition. Following the war, more and more women entered the work force while continuing their home responsibilities as wives and mothers. They were now reporting to physicians in large numbers with this same group of symptoms. A new name arose for this condition in women — *anxiety neurosis*! Unfortunately that label stuck for many years, until a physician named Barlow began to describe this group of symptoms in patients, predominantly women, who also had a sound known as a "click" heard with the stethoscope. *Barlow's syndrome* remained the popular name of the condition for quite some time. With the advent of the echocardiogram in the 1960's and the recognition of the role of the nervous system in this problem in the 1970's, the term *dysautonomia* became more frequently associated with this condition.

Although MVP syndrome is not new, our understanding of it is newer and is growing. It has been my experience that men are just as bothered by the symptoms of MVP syndrome, perhaps even more so, as are women, but fewer men are reported as having prolapse and dysautonomia. Roughly 25 percent of my patients are men. There is a simple cultural explanation for this, I think. Our culture and our society expect more stoic behavior from men. Having vague symptoms without some obvious illness is not acceptable; in fact, in some cultural circles, it is considered nonmasculine. This is grossly unfair to our brothers, but it is, nonetheless, the reality of the situation. I believe that had this condition remained one predominantly affecting males (soldier's heart) instead of females (anxiety neurosis), there would have been far more research and attention given to the subject.

Today, more and more patients are being diagnosed as having MVP. Why does this condition now seem to be reaching almost epidemic proportions? The incidence of symptoms seems to be dramatically influenced by several factors, including certain nutritional changes and the ever-increasing stress levels in our society. In our ancestor's time, the surges of adrenalin needed to escape the tiger were brief, and there was very little stress between those major events. Our lifestyle today is much more stressful on a continuous basis. Many believe that dysautonomia is so prevalent because the body must respond to stress over long periods of time, a state of being referred to as *hypervigilance.*

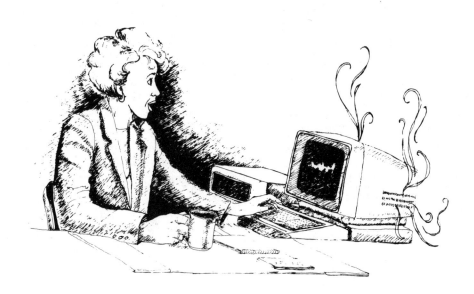

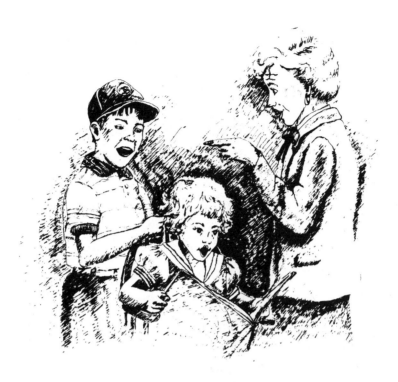

Another factor in the increased discovery of patients with MVP has been the availability of a diagnostic test known as the echocardiogram (described in detail later), first implemented in the 1960's. The echocardiogram procedure is now utilized at most medical centers. It uses sound waves to visualize the heart and its structures. It is painless and requires no injections. This test is now being performed on large numbers of patients suspected of having MVP, as well as for many other reasons, and so, more and more people are being detected with this condition.

MVP is seen in all races and on every social level. I find that many of my patients are intelligent and well-educated individuals, but I believe this reflects the greater tendency to seek health care and the higher health expectations of this particular group, rather than greater incidence in the affluent.

Some cardiology literature associates MVP with certain body types, namely the tall, slender build with long arms and fingers (Figure 1-7). My clinical impression is that this is generally true, but I have many patients who are short, round, or of average build. The description of the body type, then, is not hard and fast. Some common variations in the skeletal structure of patients are often reported. These include pectus excavatum, (sunken breast bone), and straight back.

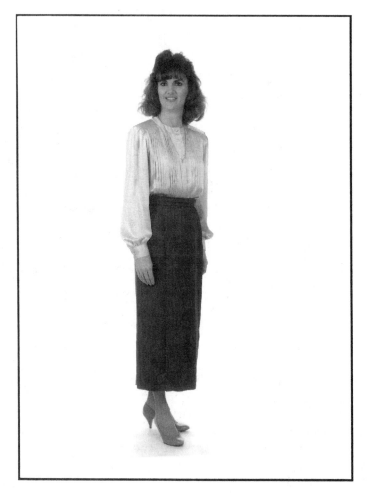

Figure 1-7

Once again this is not always the case. Another frequently occurring musculoskel-etal finding in MVP patients is the tendency to have "loose joints" (Figure 1-8). This looseness may also result in a condition known as temporo-mandibular-joint dysfunction (TMJ). TMJ may result in jaw and neck pain as well as headache be-cause of malalignment of the jaw and skull in the joint just in of front of the ear. "Loose joints" is a condition that has implications for treatment especially where exercise is concerned. These joints may be more prone to injury and, hence, safe activities must be carefully chosen.

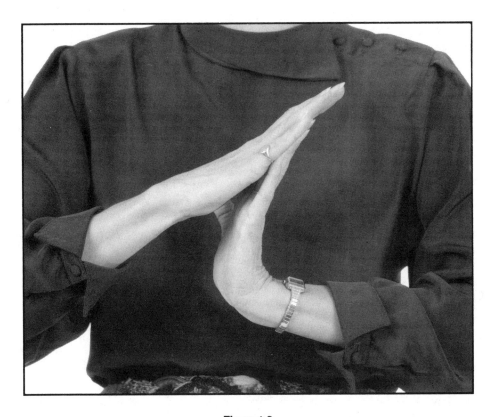

Figure 1-8

Symptoms of Mitral Valve Prolapse

Now let's take a look at an individual who shows symptoms of mitral valve prolapse and dysautonomia. She (or he) may have a normal or rapid heart rate in bed,
but the heart rate may respond inappropriately when she stands up, by accelerating
either too much or not enough. The blood vessels may respond inappropriately by
either failing to constrict properly, resulting in a fall in blood pressure, or constricting
much too rapidly, resulting in poor circulation to the hands and feet with coolness
and a bluish tint to the extremities. Both inappropriate heart rate and cold or numb
hands and feet are very common complaints among MVP patients.

Another common symptom is *chest pain*. This is one of the most frightening
symptoms of all. All the available data suggests that MVP chest pain is very different in origin from that experienced when one is having a heart attack. The pain

associated with a heart attack is a result of the heart muscle's not getting enough oxygen to meet it's needs. The chest pain in the prolapse patient may be similar in the way it feels or in its character. The chest pain is a real pain, it may be very severe, and it is frightening. It may have the same location and feel very much like a true heart attack pain, but **it is not the same**. One of the latest and probably the best known theories to date as to the origin of this pain is that when there is an imbalance in the autonomic nervous system, which controls contraction and relaxation of the chest wall muscles, the muscles of breathing, there may be inadequate relaxation between respirations. When inadequate relaxation occurs over a period of time, powerful spasms may occur in these muscles, resulting in chest pain. Another possible origin of chest pain in the patient with MVP is *esophageal reflux* — that is, the abnormal flow of stomach acid up the esophagus (the tube from the mouth to the stomach). It is believed that many patients with MVP have *esophagitis*, inflammation of the esophagus due to frequent flows of acid.

It would be foolhardy to advise people to ignore chest pain at any age. Even though the chances of having a heart attack for a younger-than-middle-age female are extremely small, it is wise to see a physician to rule out serious causes of chest pain. If the pain is found to be the result of MVP, relax, and look to later chapters for ways to control this and other symptoms. If you are a male, and some males do have prolapse and dysautonomia and chest pain, realize that your chances at all ages of having a heart attack are somewhat greater than those for a female. Chest pain should be checked out, particularly if you are beyond the age of 40, or if there is a family history of heart disease, if you smoke, or if you have any other well-known risk factors such as those listed in later chapters.

Let's look at some of the other commonly reported symptoms of individuals with MVP (Table 1-1).

Probably the most common symptom is *profound fatigue* that cannot be correlated with exercise or stress. One day a person may feel fine and have a great day; the next day she or he can barely be persuaded to get out of bed. Generally, patients report that they have never had high energy levels, that their energy level ranges from "pooped" to "super pooped," never energized. The exact reason for profound fatigue is unclear. Some recent studies suggest that people with autonomic nervous system imbalance have a tendency to have inadequate circulation to the large muscles of the arms and legs during exercise. This results in a build-up of lactic acid, as a part of Mother Nature's braking mechanism to let us know our physical limits. When lactic acid builds up to certain levels, fatigue results.

Regardless of how fatigue originates, one thing is very clear: **Fatigue breeds fatigue**. *Deconditioning* is a well-described process. It results from prolonged inactivity. Most Americans suffer from this, but more so the individual with MVP. It happens like this. Some major stress occurs that causes the MVP patient

Table 1-1. Symptoms of Mitral Valve Prolapse

Major Symptoms
    Fatigue
    Chest Pain
    Palpitations or irregular heart beat
    Migraine headache
    Anxiety
    Depression
    Panic Attacks
    Shortness of Breath
Minor Symptoms
    Neck Aches or pains
    Feeling hot or cold, not related to external temperature
    Arm or leg aches
    Shakiness
    Swelling of arms, hands, legs or feet
    Difficulty sleeping
    Backaches
    Intestinal or stomach trouble
    Difficulty with urination
    Numbness in any part of the body
    Aches or pains in hands or feet
    Fainting Spells
    Excessive perspiration or inability to perspire
    Trouble with eyes or visual disturbances
    Skin trouble or rashes
    Muscle fatigue or weakness
    Dizzy spells
    Muscular tensions
    Twitching muscles
    Poor health in general
    Excessive gas
    Bowel trouble (constipation or loose bowels)
    Hay fever or other allergies
    Trouble concentrating or memory problems

to experience chest pain, shortness of breath, and fatigue. Fear strikes. A physician is usually consulted and pronounces that the person is perfectly healthy. But the chest pain, fatigue, and shortness of breath may persist. So the person becomes less and less active. She or he may find that marketing brings on symptoms; thus, she avoids marketing. She may also notice that certain activities can result in a worsening of symptoms; hence, there is withdrawal from these. After weeks to months, some people report a virtual chair-to-bed existence. When repeated trips to the physician once again fail to show a cause, the MVP individual may either try a new physician or feel that she is going crazy. One can see the vicious cycle that develops.

A classic study done many years ago describes the deconditioning process. Several healthy young college students were put to bed for three weeks. At the end of this time, they had inappropriately high heart rates with changes in posture, their blood pressure was unstable, they felt faint, they had very little energy, and they complained of profound fatigue — classic symptoms of MVP. It took several weeks to get back to the same level of fitness they had enjoyed prior to the experiment. Is this message beginning to be clear? Fatigue is only one part of a vicious cycle that can be set up in the MVP patient. The goal of patients with MVP is to break this cycle by whatever means available and slowly restore the individual to his or her previous level of fitness, if not better. This is done by modifying several factors in the individual's life: diet, exercise, and mental attitude. Each of these will be covered in detail in later chapters.

Another common symptom is the *inability to think clearly*. This is most disturbing, and as one intelligent MVP patient said, this may be one of the most upsetting symptoms of all. MVP patients in this condition are very concerned that they are losing their mental faculties. The exact reasons for the "spaced out" feelings are not completely clear. Sometimes the feelings come from medications that are used in an attempt to regulate the autonomic nervous system. At other times, deconditioning may play a role. Just as the body does not tolerate being off its feet very well, as demonstrated by the college students placed on bed rest, neither does the nervous system tolerate a lack of physical activity at whatever level. Finally, MVP symptoms can be very disturbing, often completely occupying a person's thinking hour after hour, day in and day out. When that is the case, all objectivity is lost, and one tends to dwell on bodily processes excessively. We refer to this as *somatic preoccupation*. This simply means enhanced awareness of bodily functions. It does not mean that one is neurotic or that the symptoms are "all in your head." It says, rather, that a vicious cycle is going on in your body and life over which you have very little, if any, control. This is upsetting and even depressing. Yes, depressing. Is it any wonder that feeling lousy day in and day out, the MVP patient gets depressed? The important thing to remember is that for you, the MVP patient, this need not go on forever! There are ways out of this vicious cycle that will once again return your destiny to your hands and get you back in reasonable physical condition. When this happens, the "fuzzy head" usually clears, as does the depression. There. I have said it! **You are not crazy!** Of course, there are some neurotic MVP people; but, there are also neurotic non-MVP folks. It's like apples and oranges. MVP and neurosis are not the same thing.

Another frequently mentioned symptom is *irritable bowel syndrome,* chronic constipation or diarrhea, which can be a very worrisome problem. I recently had a patient who had not been out to dinner or on a vacation for two years because of fear of sudden diarrhea that would cause her to soil her clothes. Ulcers also are reported, most often in young females.

Sleep problems are also associated with MVP syndrome. Both the inability to fall asleep and problems staying asleep are common. Another very disturbing symptom associated with sleep is the nocturnal panic attack — that is, awakening in the middle of the night feeling like you are smothering or with rapid heartbeat and shortness of breath. This will be discussed further in the chapter on anxiety and panic. Some of the medications commonly used to treat MVP in the past often made the sleep problems worse.

There are a number of other symptoms that many people report. Not every person with MVP will have every symptom, but an amazing number of similarities can be found. Many people report *palpitations*, a fluttering sensation in the chest that may be the result of rapid heartbeats or extra early heartbeats. As previously mentioned, there are patients who have serious irregularities in the heart rhythm that should be treated, but these conditions are very rare. Most MVP patients have extra heartbeats that are of absolutely no consequence. It is not uncommon for the MVP patient to report *dizziness*, *shakiness*, *shortness of breath*, *muscle fatigue*, and *frequent headaches*, to name just a few of the symptoms.

A study of my last 300 patients shows that the vast majority of them have more than one symptom but that the major reason for seeking treatment can usually be one of the five symptoms as shown in Figure 1-9. Fatigue is by far the most common and worrisome complaint followed by palpitations, chest pain, panic attacks, and headache. Other symptoms, such as irritable bowel and dizziness, are not uncommon but are usually not the symptom that makes patients seek treatment.

Some interesting research suggests that people with dysautonomia have *extremely sensitive nervous systems*. This does not mean that they are emotionally sensitive, although they may be that also. Rather, the nervous system is sensitive to all the stimulation put to it — sights, sounds, touch, posture, temperature, and all stresses that affect us in our daily life. The dysautonomic patient seems to perceive these stimuli more intensely than the average person. For example, the average person may smell a strong chemical and find it offensive. The dysautonomic person may be so sensitive to the same chemical odor that she or he may develop a migraine headache. Another example is the sense of touch, feeling, or pressure. The MVP patient is always surprised to hear that the average person usually cannot feel his or her own heartbeat unless vigorously exercising or suddenly frightened. In contrast, the MVP patients can almost always feel their heartbeat, even at rest. They can also usually feel the blood flow in the arteries on the side of the head. Average persons cannot, unless they put their head on a pillow in just a certain way. Dysautonomic patients may report with alarm that at night while nearly asleep, they stop breathing for periods of time, and then take a deep breath. Everyone does this! The average person is simply not aware of it. MVP patients report that when they climb stairs, they are aware of a strong heartbeat, and breathe very hard; everyone does, but the rest of the world is simply not aware of it. Persons without MVP also have a wide range in their heart rate during the day as well as during various activities, but they simply do not sit with their finger on their pulse! In later chapters, signs and symptoms to be attended to will be distinguished from those to be ignored. If you are aware of irregular heartbeats or palpitations, once your physician

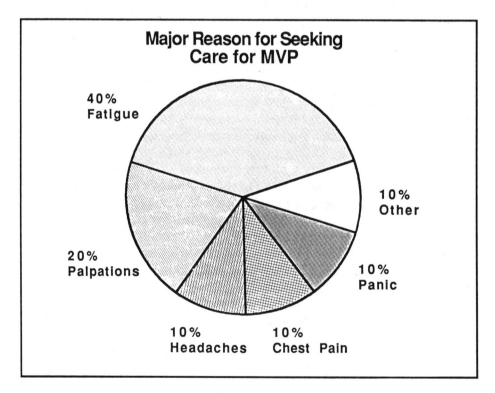

Figure 1-9

has determined that there is nothing to worry about, you will need to begin to desensitize yourself to some of these sensations.

Migraine headaches are frequently reported by MVP patients. They are thought to be due to sensitive blood vessels under the control of the autonomic nervous system. Generally, migraine headaches are due to either abnormal dilation of blood vessels or constriction of blood vessels within the brain. Fortunately, when the entire body is brought back into balance with a comprehensive program for prolapse patients, the headaches become less frequent and often, less severe.

MVP patients frequently report shortness of breath with very mild activity. The cause may be complex, but once again, the symptom may be attributed to the fact that the muscles of breathing or respiration are under the control of the autonomic nervous system. Any imbalance in this system could result in rapid or irregular breathing or respirations. I believe, however, that the primary cause of shortness of breath is that the MVP patient has undergone deconditioning. As mentioned before, some symptoms result from the lack of activity that begins the deconditioning process. The college students previously mentioned, when put to bed for just three weeks, became very short of breath with only mild exertion for at least four to six weeks after their return to activity. Imagine for a moment that the typical prolapse patient has been troubled with symptoms and virtually incapacitated for several months or even years. She or he is profoundly deconditioned. The deconditioning results in unstable blood pressure, somewhat lower-than-normal circulating blood volume, marked fatigue, inappropriate heart rates, and shortness of breath. These are exactly the same symptoms that most patients report with MVP. Where do the symptoms associated with MVP stop and those of deconditioning begin? The vicious cycle must be broken and the deconditioning reversed before it is possible to say which symptoms are the result of MVP alone.

Many MVP patients report having "spells." With careful questioning, these can be identified as anxiety or panic attacks. Many of our patients do not like the term "panic attack," because it implies a neurotic origin. Let me assure you that panic attacks have a biochemical basis. Numerous scientific studies have proven this. Panic attacks can be extremely uncomfortable and very frightening and, in fact, warrant a separate chapter later in the book. But let me say here that they are controllable and that most patients who complete our program overcome these attacks.

It is not uncommon for women with prolapse to report very tender breasts prior to their menstrual periods, and some even give a history of having been diagnosed with fibrocystic breast disease, a tendency for painful, lumpy breasts. Once again, the exact link is unknown, but when women become involved in the diet and exercise program outlined in this book, they report that the pain in their breasts subsides dramatically.

Premenstrual syndrome (PMS) is a topic very much in vogue today. It has been given a lot of attention in newspapers, books, journals, and women's magazines.

When questioned, about 80 percent of our patients say that they suffer from some or all of the symptoms of premenstrual syndrome, including problem swelling, mood swings, abdominal pain, and personality changes. It is not yet clear whether dysautonomia indeed plays a role in PMS, or whether, as previously mentioned, our patients are merely more in tune and aware of changes in their own bodies than the average person. We hope that our research will answer some of these questions.

Many of my patients report a history of allergies. This is a very interesting association and has some real promise for research in the future. The allergy most often reported by prolapse patients is one to yeast. Yeast is a very common allergen and it is difficult to avoid. It is found on the skin of every living organism, and a few foods such as vinegar and alcoholic beverages, are absolutely loaded with yeast. Interestingly, most dysautonomic patients report that they are very sensitive to all alcohol, and some are unable to tolerate even a glass of wine. This is thought to be due to both their sensitivity to yeast in the alcohol and their supersensitive nervous system.

If you are troubled by allergies, there is no substitute for being seen by a good allergist and getting that problem straightened out. Yeast sensitivity tends to be a problem in patients who have at some time taken large doses of antibiotics to treat an infection. Antibiotics allow yeast to grow unchecked in the body. Women using birth control pills are more likely to develop yeast infections than those who don't take them. Many female prolapse patients report frequent vaginal yeast infections.

One of the most exciting areas of research in mitral valve prolapse is elucidating the biochemical basis for many of the symptoms. Many researchers believe that although at least 10 percent of the population has MVP, the occurrence of the symptoms must be biochemically triggered. One reason this is thought to be true, is that at least 95 percent of the patients seen can report a precipitating event of some kind. This could be an emotional stress, such as death of a loved one, divorce, or a new job. Or, it could be great physical stress, such as an accident, surgery, a severe viral illness, flu, or severe illness, that immediately precedes the onset of symptoms. We believe that certain predictable chemical events follow great stress of any kind.

Many MVP patients have been previously labeled as hypoglycemic (having low blood sugar), usually incorrectly. The symptoms of hypoglycemia are very similar to the most common prolapse symptoms, such as fatigue, shakiness associated with hunger, and the tendency to have a "sweet tooth." This will be further discussed in the chapter on diet. But, an interesting bit of information is that approximately 80 percent of female patients admitted to a major teaching hospital recently with the label "hypoglycemic" were found to have mitral valve prolapse and dysautonomia, and with careful testing were found not to be truly hypoglycemic.

However, many patients have hypoglycemia as part of their mitral valve prolapse syndrome.

It is common for patients to come to me having been told that they had another condition, such as hyperventilation syndrome (panic attacks), anxiety states (panic attacks), depression (due to lack of energy), and even thyroid dysfunction (the tendency to gain or loose weight). With careful diagnostic testing these other diagnosis are often ruled out in favor of MVP and dysautonomia.

Confused Conditions

- Hypoglycemia

- Anxiety State

- Hyperventilation

- Depression

- Premenstrual Syndrome

- Thyroid Dysfunction

Diagnosis of Mitral Valve Prolapse

You may be getting the impression that the MVP syndrome is complex. It is. You may say "I often feel fatigued, and sometimes I feel spaced out. Could I have mitral valve prolapse syndrome? How do I tell?" Usually, a physician listening to your beating heart can hear a special sound known as a *click*, made by the mitral valve when it billows back into the upper chamber of the heart. Some people with MVP also have a very quiet *heart murmur*, a sound created when a small amount of blood leaks backward through the floppy valve. Upon detecting a click or a murmur, your doctor may order a test known as an echocardiogram — a test that uses sound waves to detect abnormalities of the heart (Figure 1-10). Usually this test is enough to establish whether an individual has mitral valve prolapse.

The diagnosis of MVP syndrome is a clinical diagnosis. That is, the diagnosis is made from the total complex of symptoms and findings on physical examination. For example a physician diagnoses measles based on symptoms and physical exam; that is a clinical diagnosis and is not made on the basis of a special blood test or other types of tests, but from clinical criteria alone. More detailed tests, such as cardiac catheterization are usually not necessary to diagnose MVP syndrome. Cardiac catheterization is a procedure that utilizes a catheter, which is introduced into a blood vessel and advanced to the heart, at which time contrast material is injected to visualize the heart structures. The only time that such a procedure would be recommended is if a more complicated problem needed to be ruled out. Occasionally, patients who have a strong family history of heart disease, or patients who are above the age of 40 to 45 years and are suffering chest pain, must have a cardiac catheterization to make sure that they do not have more serious causes for their pain.

What about dysautonomia? How can you tell whether you have that? The diagnosis of dysautonomia is often much more difficult than the MVP diagnosis. Your physician may suspect dysautonomia if you have MVP. If so, he or she may recommend medication. The diagnosis of dysautonomia is also a clinical diagnosis, based on symptoms and objective findings on examination. There are only two or three centers in the United States that have specialized laboratories designed to look at the function of the autonomic nervous system. The test for dysautonomia

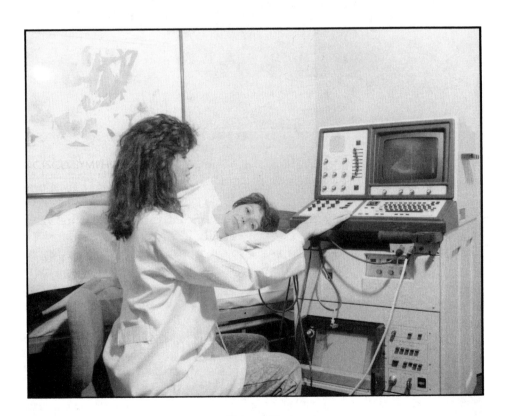

Figure 1-10

involves a series of *noninvasive* procedures; that is, the tests do not use needles or catheters, or cause pain. A tilt table is utilized that evaluates a patient in both reclining and standing positions (Figure 1-11); other specialized equipment reflects the function of the autonomic nervous system during various simple maneuvers such as deep breathing. A patient's heart rate is evaluated, and changes in heart rate with the changes in posture also reflect the function of the autonomic nervous system. One's blood pressure and cardiac output (the amount of blood that the heart actually pumps out) may also evaluated.

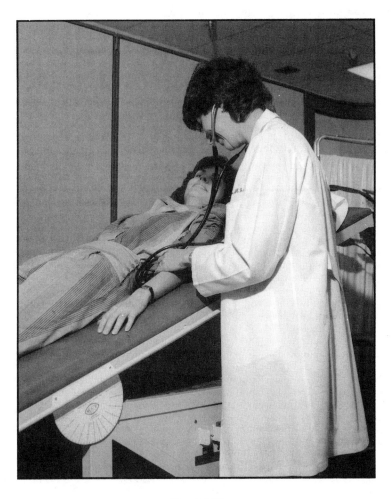

Figure 1-11

With the results of these tests, a determination is made as to the nature of the imbalance of the autonomic nervous system. Therapy that is appropriate to the particular type of imbalance can then be chosen, and later the patient may be retested to evaluate progress. Remember that one can have MVP with dysautonomia and MVP without dysautonomia, but quite often they occur together (Figure 1-12).

Let me share with you some patient studies as examples. I have seen patients from all over the country, and indeed, all over the world. If you are a patient of mine, you may recognize yourself. All of the names have been changed though. And all circumstances have been altered so that no one else will recognize you. I have already mentioned my friend Jane. Jane felt perfectly well until four years ago, prior to admission to the hospital. She had two grown children, and had suffered only the usual colds and flu without serious illness or injury. Four years ago she noticed extreme fatigue and a rather bluish tint to her extremities, which were icy cold. She was diagnosed as having hypoglycemia (low blood sugar) and Raynaud's syndrome (poor circulation to the hands and feet). For the next four years she followed a high-protein diet and kept her hands and feet well wrapped but her progress was only fair. She had undergone multiple hospitalizations in an attempt to pinpoint her problem and psychiatric care had been suggested by more than one physician. When I met Jane, she was depressed and reluctant to share her roller-

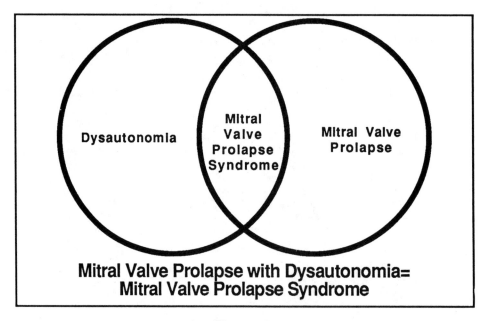

Figure 1-12

coaster history. She warmed immediately when she found out that she was not alone, that I had numerous patients with the same problems. In getting to know Jane, I found her to be one of the most charming, emotionally stable individuals I had ever met. When I visited her in the hospital I would leave the room feeling better because of her ability to always find something nice to say. She began the diet and exercise program as well as some medications prescribed by her physician. A couple of months later she reported that she was feeling wonderful, walking every day, and doing just "peachy," to use her word. Unfortunately, she had a rather difficult time with some dental work and had a major setback that took her months to get over. Jane's positive mental attitude and her supportive family enabled her to come back to the active world. She still has setbacks from time to time, but her course is plotted in a very positive direction.

Another of my patients is an extremely active physician's wife who was completely well until the birth of her last child, about two years ago. She had previously been a jogger, but for the last several months, she had been unable to keep up with her daily activities and was profoundly fatigued. She also experienced frightening chest pain and frequent migraine headaches. The constant fatigue rendered her unable to maintain her busy social schedule and was causing marital problems. She began our diet and exercise program and was feeling much better, without the need for medication of any sort.

Another patient in my files is a tragic 25-year-old woman whom I saw only a few weeks ago. She also had the onset of her symptoms following the birth of a second child. Her major symptom was profound fatigue. Her chest pain was minimal, but she did complain of rapid heartbeat. She had been sent from one small-town physician to another without finding an answer. Finally, in desperation, she followed the advice of one of these physicians and was hospitalized for psychiatric care. She underwent several electroshock treatments and was released. A friend of ours recommended that she come to see me for an evaluation, and, sure enough, she had MVP and marked dysautonomia. I might mention that my impression of this woman was that she was indeed depressed. I would be, too, if I had been tired and defeated for two years. With diet and exercise and small amounts of medication, her lifestyle has improved dramatically already.

Just to present a different sort of case, I will tell you about Gertrude. She was a middle-aged nurse with the most bizarre symptoms I had ever heard. When I asked her what sorts of things brought on her symptoms, she replied that riding in a car did it (not so unusual). Her solution was to have her husband watch the odometer, pull off the road every mile exactly, shut off the motor and sit for exactly two minutes, then proceed. I thought this was a little compulsive, but nevertheless continued with the interview. The thing that she said bothered her heart the most was when she washed her bottom in the bathtub! I tried not to giggle, and I asked her how she managed to solve this problem, because she was obviously a well-groomed, nice-looking lady. She told me that her husband had been washing her bottom for the last five years. This lady had prolapse, but obviously that was not her major problem. I suggested that she see a psychiatrist. I use this case to point out the fact that there is neurosis and there is MVP. They are not the same thing, nor are they mutually exclusive. In short, there is no relationship.

Summing Up

In summary, MVP syndrome is a combination of symptoms that accompanies a structural variation of the heart valve. Each patient is different, and although there are numerous similarities, no two people exhibit exactly the same set of symptoms. Symptoms may vary from hour to hour, day to day, or week to week. A person may feel fine on Monday, wiped out on Tuesday, and terrific on Wednesday. (A more common scenario for the MVP patient is fair on Monday, lousy on Tuesday, and so-so on Thursday).

The MVP syndrome is an extremely common condition. It has been described by authors for generations. It is not new; it is just that our ways of diagnosis and treatment are new. It is not a life-threatening condition, but may be lifestyle threatening if the symptoms are so uncomfortable and frightening that a person cannot cope with them. No two patients have the same symptoms or the same severity of symptoms. The only thing that can be said for all prolapse patients is that there are a number of things they can all do to help themselves feel better, including proper diet, exercise, and positive mental attitude.

2 The Impact of Mitral Valve Prolapse on Relationships

MVP can often take its toll on our everyday relationships, both at home and at work — in a marriage, for example. When you marry, you have an unwritten contract as to the role of the individuals involved. Typically,the male will earn a living, take out the trash, do other "masculine" endeavors and will be supportive, loving, and entertaining. The female is expected, perhaps, to work to help support the family and to be a loving mother, an affectionate wife, a charming hostess, and a good friend to all. When symptoms of mitral valve prolapse appear and persist for prolonged periods of time, the unwritten contract that was agreed upon before the marriage changes. Suddenly the MVP partner is no longer fulfilling his or her part of the bargain. This can lead to devastating marital problems. Even the most supportive, loving partner has a limit to the amount of support he or she they can give in the absence of information about what the problem is.

In the past few years I have had the opportunity to counsel hundreds of couples whose relationships were beginning to be affected by MVP. The approach to this problem is not always easy. Initially I begin the education process with the spouse the same way I do with the patients — to help him or her understand what the problem is, what the source of the symptoms is, and what types of symptoms can be expected. I then go into great detail about the lifestyle modifications that are necessary to stabilize the condition, and I emphasize that the support of the spouse is essential in maintaining such a balance.

It is difficult for me to evaluate the interactions of MVP patients with those around them. Often, because patients have been symptomatic for a long time, they have come to view themselves as "sick" people. They have established their relationships in a very dependent fashion. When a relationship is established in such a way, it is often very difficult to make changes in that relationship, even if all agree that they would be for the better. Unfortunately, a few patients with mitral valve prolapse syndrome get into a pattern of manipulating the people around them through the use of their symptoms. They form the unhealthy habit of using their symptoms as an excuse for virtually everything, from not pulling their share of the work around the house, to not being satisfied with their job, to not being the type of spouse their mate expects them to be. This is not the rule, and these patients represent an extreme, but the tendency when you have a problem over a prolonged period of time is to become the dependent partner. Likewise, the partner without MVP takes on the role of the protector and nurturer, a role that may be somewhat threatened when the patient begins to feel better, more assertive, and more capable in the world.

For anyone in this situation, I would recommend the services of a professional counselor — a clinical psychologist, a marriage counselor, or some other professional individual with a knowledge of MVP, as well as marital counseling skills. Sometimes taking a close look at your interpersonal relationships is very difficult and somewhat painful. But like many other difficult activities in life, it is usually worth the pain and the effort it requires.

MVP and the Job

Just like the marital relationship, relationships on the job require an unwritten and sometimes a written contract about what activities the employee will perform, during what hours, for how many days a week, and so on. When symptoms of the mitral valve prolapse syndrome come along, often the patient is unable to fulfill his or her part of the bargain. Absences and tardiness are very frequent. Generally poor performance can result in poor job relationships. Most of us need to work to feed ourselves and provide for our families. The MVP patient must protect his or her job relationship and understand that the employer has every right to expect certain activities. If you have MVP symptoms, you should make every effort to fulfill your obligations to your employer.

I am often asked by patients whether or not they should say on a pre-employment health questionnaire that they have a heart murmur and have problems with MVP. This is a very difficult question to answer. The MVP syndrome has recently received a great deal of attention, and there are probably certain employers who would be somewhat hesitant to hire an individual if they thought there was going to be a chronic health problem. In a few years we hope to have educated the public to realize that mitral valve prolapse syndrome is merely a variant of the normal condition and that most people who have it are perfectly capable of fulfilling their work obligations as well as anyone else. In fact, patients with MVP who follow very healthful lifestyles to improve symptoms tends to drink less, be healthier, and have fewer health problems than the general population. The reason for this is that the MVP patient's body cannot tolerate the abuses that many other individuals can heap upon themselves for years before their bodies start to break down.

I would give the same advice to an MVP patient applying for insurance. I would never advise anyone to conceal information regarding health history, and I believe that insurance carriers now are wise enough to realize that MVP is a variant and that most people with MVP are never going to cost them any more than the general population, and may well cost them less.

You and the Rest of the World

MVP patients are mothers, fathers, brothers, sisters, sons, daughters, and friends. It is impossible to have severe, prolonged symptoms such as those sometimes seen with MVP and not have some of these relationships change. For this reason, I think it is often very valuable for MVP patients to have professional counseling to enable them to find the skills to meet these problems head on and not allow their symptoms to interfere with the interpersonal relationships that we all need in our daily lives for richness and for fulfillment.

Special effort must be made to maintain the health of the parent-child relationship. When a mother has the mitral valve prolapse syndrome and prolonged symptoms, her small children may suffer. They may come to see their mother as a "sick person." Children often feel guilty when a parent is ill, not realizing that they are in no way to blame for their parent's condition. They may feel guilty for watching television or playing loudly, or indulging in other typical childhood activities that may annoy the symptomatic parent. Over a prolonged period of time, this can be damaging to the child and to the parent-child relationship. The parent with MVP should make every effort to budget time carefully and spend as much good-quality time with the children as possible.

Do MVP patients make good friends? Observing the support groups for panic attack patients and other groups, I have seen many MVP patients become extremely good friends to one another. They can offer a unique kind of support because they do truly understand. MVP patients' friends who do not have prolapse often find it difficult to understand the situation, as spouses do. In friendship as in a marital or job relationship, your friend has a right to expect that you will be there to meet his or her needs on occasion, as well as the other way around. When a mitral valve prolapse patient seems to be constantly complaining or never feeling like going out, friendships can suffer. As with all other relationships, realize that the other person has needs, too. No relationship can be a one-way street. Realizing this will enable MVP patients to think about the needs of the other individuals in their lives and at least periodically try to meet these needs rather than constantly focusing on their own problems.

Often my MVP patients are very intelligent people who have accurate insight into their own behavior and that of those around them. They feel a great deal of guilt at their inability to meet the needs of their family and friends. This can become a severe problem that leads to depression. To these people, I would once again reiterate the importance of a positive mental attitude and undertaking a comprehensive program to stabilize the situation. Depression can result in a "yesbut" response to this kind of suggestion. I will use this term many times in this book. It defines the individual that replies "yes, but" any time a new suggestion is made. They seem to have a long list of reasons why they can't try something new. When we are depressed, it is very difficult to be hopeful. Thus, it is very hard to undertake a difficult program with enough resolve to stick to it. In cases like this, group support sessions are invaluable.

As previously mentioned, when a person feels lousy for a prolonged period of time, there is a great tendency to focus inward on one's self and one's own symptoms. I would caution you, the MVP patient, to try to turn your attention outward to the loved ones around you, to try to meet their needs, and to avoid the unhealthy focus on your own personal problems. MVP need not stand in the way of living and loving.

3 You and Your Physician

This chapter was extremely difficult to write. I believe that some of the information contained in this chapter, however, is some of the most useful in the entire book. I work every day with physicians and I am married to a wonderful physician. I have been fortunate to work with a number of excellent physicians who are very knowledgeable and compassionate individuals. I believe that there are many such physicians throughout the country, but the difficult task is locating them. I realize that some of what I say in this chapter could subject me to a great deal of criticism from my physician colleagues. But I believe that the information presented is critical to the overall understanding of this problem.

Most of my patients report varying degrees of difficulty in past experiences with physicians. Some were fortunate in that they were diagnosed and sent to the MVP Center rather quickly. Most, however, have spent a great deal of time trying to find out what is wrong with them. Many have seen numerous physicians. Commonly they report that their symptoms have received little, if any, attention. Worse are the reports that they have been openly ridiculed or shamed for their symptoms. I have yet to have a patient referred to me who felt that she or he had been given adequate information regarding MVP — what it is, its implications for lifestyle, ways to help solve the problem, diet, exercise, and so forth. It is very difficult for me to defend this type of treatment, or lack of it, and yet I believe I do need to say a few words in defense of the majority of well-meaning physicians in practice today. There is very little information in the professional literature about the complexity of symptoms experienced by the MVP patient. But there is plenty of literature that speaks to the benign (not serious) nature of the problem. It is for this reason, I am sure, that a number of physicians simply do not understand the extent of the problem.

During their long years of education, physicians are taught to question everything and to depend on well-proven facts. They are extremely skeptical of new "hot items" that are not thoroughly researched. There is, as I have said, very little information in the literature regarding the symptoms of MVP and their complex interaction with the autonomic nervous system. There is even less information about successful methods of treatment. In addition, several rather prominent authorities in the field of cardiovascular pathology (diseases) do not believe that many of the symptoms have any basis other than in the patient's mind. One such physician came to this area not long ago as a visiting professor. He had been doing some of the most highly respected long-term work about the natural history of MVP, that is, what happens to people with MVP without treatment. His studies are the ones I am reporting when I say that the MVP patient has the same life expectancy as the general population. Once when he was addressing a rather large gathering of physicians and was asked about the symptoms suffered by patients with MVP, he replied that it was all hogwash. He believed that some patients could experience palpitations, that is fluttering of the heartbeats, or even chest pain, but that the other symptoms were just a sign of neurosis. He believed that the anxiety level was extremely high in these patients and that generally they enjoyed what was referred to as NIH, neurotic ill health. There is no way to tell you how I felt sitting there listening to him — anger, rage, would not begin to describe my feelings. What made it worse was that the room was filled with eager, young physicians beginning to form their opinions, about various things and they were being influenced by him. I was absolutely livid.

As I have already mentioned, I believe that the slight imbalance in the autonomic nervous system often associated with MVP can indeed account for many of the symptoms experienced by the MVP patient. I also believe that deconditioning can then come into play. And I also have to believe that when a person has some symptom, regardless of what it is, sees a physician, and is told that there is "an abnormality in your heart," that person suffers anxiety. I know from personal experience with my patients how detrimental anxiety can be. Like deconditioning, anxiety can set up a vicious cycle and can dramatically interfere with a person's recovery. When these factors are combined — autonomic nervous system imbalance, deconditioning, and anxiety — a terrible cycle is introduced. Several years later, when a person finally comes to see me, I have to be honest and admit that I frequently have a difficult time sorting out which problem is from which source.

The body is a wondrous system; it is infinitely complicated. God has given us numerous back-up systems and defense mechanisms. I also believe that the mind is far more powerful than we have yet discovered. We already know that stress can play a major role in peptic ulcer disease, colitis, heart disease, and high blood pressure. A number of individuals are studying the role of stress on MVP syndrome. Remember, not only does stress begin some of these diseases, but once established, the diseases themselves can induce even more stress. One of my primary goals is to investigate these complicated interactions, Every patient I see fills out an extensive questionnaire, undergoes numerous diagnostic procedures, and is re-evaluated periodically. All of this information is fed into computer systems for analysis. We hope to publish this information and to spread the word to physicians throughout the country. Physicians want to practice medicine based on relationships that can be seen and proven. The MVP-stress-deconditioning relationship has not been fully elucidated and has not yet received widespread acceptance. We hope this will change in the next few years.

Let me share with you why I believe there is such a negative mind set among many physicians dealing with MVP patients. Remember the story of my patient whose husband had been washing her bottom for five years? How did this woman's problems begin? I really don't know. It is possible that she had been rather unstable all of her life. I assure you that most if not all of the physicians who came into contact with this woman were thereafter convinced that MVP was synonymous with neurosis. She was an extreme case. The usual patient has some symptom — fatigue, chest pain, palpitations, or whatever. She may see one physician or she may see several without finding any answers about what is wrong with her. Physicians are human, and they believe what they can see — she has absolutely nothing wrong with her by physical examination or by any of the commonly available tests that would explain her symptoms. Her physician gets frustrated. He has an office full of patients with illnesses that he is familiar with and that he can treat. He can even become resentful of the amount of time taken up by this patient who has absolutely nothing that he can put his finger on. Many physicians do not like to have their diagnoses or orders questioned. The MVP patient seems to question everything. This is a reflection of anxiety and a desperate attempt to gain reassurance and more information about the problem. A few physicians are hung up in the authority role and do not appreciate it when a patient tries to assume responsibility for his or her own health or asks intelligent questions. These few are not for you. When the physician becomes impatient with the MVP patient's lack of progress, or feels that a not-so-serious condition is occupying an unusually large amount of time, he or she may transfer the patient to someone else — a specialist such as a cardiologist, psychiatrist, or neurologist. (Let me quickly say that I do not think that every referral to a psychiatrist is bad. There is more discussion of this later.)

If the patient is lucky and within the first three or four physicians visited the MVP problem is discovered, he or she is usually told that this condition "involves the heart," and, "Don't worry." Any fool knows that the heart is an absolutely vital organ and that a problem with this organ can be life-threatening. Thus, the "Don't worry" falls on deaf ears. I believe that the anxiety component of MVP syndrome would be dramatically altered if at this point the physician would take the time to explain the nature of the condition and give some much needed reassurance to the patient. Unfortunately until now there had been nothing in print that patients could take home and read. There was nothing they could show their families that would explain their sometimes unusual behavior or tell the families what could be done to support them. Worse yet, this lack of information can make the patients feel helpless and not in control of their own bodies. This fosters dependence on the physician that, I can assure you, the physician will not be very happy about later on. Fear can do some rather striking things to the body that can be very detrimental over time.

Physicians in our country are wonderfully trained, yet most would tell you that the hectic pace of medical school does not allow much time for instruction in the behavioral sciences. Medical students have told me that they have so much to learn in their really high-powered science courses, that they do not want to "waste their hours" on "all of that psychological stuff," — even when they realize that someday they will need those pieces of information. Many physicians in the United States believe that all health problems are ultimately resolved with a pill, surgery, time, or death. They receive very little training in conditions that do not respond so neatly and do not fit into a preconceived slot. Physicians in other countries, European countries, for example, have long recognized the needs of people for good nutrition, exercise, and so on, and have done some really good work to elucidate the role of dietary modifications in MVP patients. In this country we seem to want a quick fix. This is a symptom of our entire society. When patients first see their physician for some symptom of prolapse, they expect that the doctor can give them a pill or a potion and make them better instantly. *This is an unrealistic expectation.* You must take responsibility for your own health. There is only so much that any physician can do for the MVP patients. The rest of their health care is in their own hands. It is not easy. It is hard work to get yourself in good shape and maintain good health. I have said that the body is a wonderful system with all sorts of built-in mechanisms for self-defense. It allows us to abuse it by overeating, smoking, and lack of exercise for example. But for the mitral valve prolapse patient, it becomes very important to take care of yourself. Like anyone else, you are responsible for your own health. There are some times when you should seek the care of your physician and to not do so would be foolhardy, but on a day-to-day basis you are in charge of your own health.

Do Not Turn Off Your Physician

Although there are times when I believe it is appropriate to seek the opinion or care of another physician, for the most part, that does not solve the problem. Usually, you have to get along with the physician that you have. The first of Frederickson's Laws — you will hear more of them throughout the book — is "Do not turn off your physician." For this reason I have listed below behavior that "turns off," or annoys physicians. You may find this list amusing, and I hope that you do, but the reason for presenting the list is to help you see by contrast ways to form a *good* relationship with your physician. Later in the chapter I have given you a list of ways to help form this kind of a bond.

Ways To Turn Off Your Physician

1. Stop by the office without an appointment to ask questions or to be seen.

2. Call him or her at home to discuss your problem. You get extra points if you call late at night.

3. Bring to your appointment a three page (or longer) list of your symptoms.

4. Alter your own medication schedule as you see the need.

5. Suggest other methods of treatment that he or she may want to try, for example, the treatment used on your friend with a similar condition.

6. Suggest that he or she read an article in your monthly women's magazine about MVP.

7. Be late for appointments.

8. Make sure your appearance does not match your reported symptoms; that is, while telling him that you have been absolutely unable to function, you are wiped out, and you feel terrible, look absolutely smashing, perfectly groomed, with perfect makeup.

9. Make your own diagnosis.

10. Say "Yes but ..." to his every suggestion.

11. Be aggressive and hostile. Get angry at your physician because he or she cannot help you.

12. Suggest that he or she read this book.

As you can see from this list, there are a number of things patients commonly do that physicians find offensive. This is by no means a complete list — only a start. For each entry, think of a better way to interact with your physician. For example, *don't* drop by the office and interrupt his or her schedule, expecting to be seen. Remember that your physician has numerous other patients — most with conditions easier to see and understand than yours. Don't assume that he or she has all the time in the world for you. If you have been fortunate and have a physician who is very understanding and has spent a great deal of time reassuring you about MVP and the related symptoms, don't constantly seek reassurance.

Be patient. When your physician puts you on medication, don't assume that you will feel better tomorrow. It took a great deal of time, perhaps months or years, to get into the condition you are in today. It is unrealistic to expect that any pill or any program is going to make you better overnight. Likewise, if you are not put on medication and you only follow the guidelines in this book, don't assume that you will feel better tomorrow. It usually takes months or even years for the MVP patient to get into perfect condition. To expect overnight wellness is absolutely unrealistic. Don't even expect steady improvement. There will be setbacks. Sometimes your physician may need to readjust or even change your medication. This is not uncommon. I try to stabilize patients using diet, exercise, and reassurance alone, without resorting to medication. But this is not always possible. Some patients have extremely uncomfortable symptoms that make it impossible for them to exercise or follow the rest of the program. These patients have to be put on medication immediately. Later in the book I have included a list of medications frequently used in treating MVP patients. Please don't look at the list and make suggestions to your doctor. The purpose of the list is merely to familiarize you with some of the approaches used with the prolapse patient, not to allow you to prescribe for yourself. I am learning every day about this condition. Many researchers are beginning to be interested in investigating the many presentations of MVP. New medications and new approaches are constantly being tried. We hope that by the time this book is in print, we will have even more answers to the problem than we do today.

Physicians are human. There is a limit to the patience of even the kindest, most compassionate, most saintly physician. This is not to say that you must put on a false front or claim to be better when you are not. Just avoid unrealistic expectations. Also, remember that you are responsible for a large part of your treatment — diet, exercise, and positive mental attitude. Your physician cannot do it without your help.

Stabilizing the Doctor-Patient Relationship

In contrast to the list provided earlier in the chapter, here are some ways to help make the doctor-patient relationship work well for you:

How To Maintain A Relationship with Your Physician

1. Be honest with your physician and yourself.

2. When you need to see your physician, make an appointment. If you need to call his office for advice, speak with the nurse if possible and be as brief as you can.

3. Be concise when you are with your physician. Organize your thoughts, but don't bring lengthy notes.

4. Take your medication as prescribed. Many medications may actually make you feel somewhat worse before you start feeling better. Your physician prescribed your medication for a reason. Take it as directed.

5. Take responsibility for your health. Your physician cannot maintain your diet, exercise, and positive mental attitude. You must provide these for yourself.

6. Don't be a yesbut! Be open to new suggestions.

7. Discuss problems openly and honestly with your physician before entertaining the idea of changing physicians.

8. Practice assertive behavior. Take an assertiveness training course.

9. Be on time for your appointments. If you must miss an appointment, call and cancel.

10. Maintain your well-groomed appearance, but be aware that if you look dazzling, you might not be taken seriously.

11. Let the physician do the diagnosing.

12. Be assertive, but avoid aggressive or hostile outburst, regardless of how you feel.

If you already have a physician and your relationship is not what you would like it to be, you must make some changes. Take a look at your former interactions. Has he or she tended to lose patience with you? Have you really expected too much? Do you have a good enough relationship that he or she would be open to new information such as "I've been trying this diet that has really been of help to me. Can I tell you about it?." In future interactions try to be aware of the way he or she may be feeling so that you can avoid some of the negative interactions. A good patient-physician relationship is very important to the MVP patient, as it is to everyone in need of health care. As with all relationships, it may require some work.

Another one of Frederickson's Laws is "Be honest." Honesty with your physician and with yourself will go a long way in stabilizing your relationship. I have already mentioned that many of my patients are almost ashamed of their unusual symptoms. They may put on a false front of pretending to be better, when in fact, they are not. Or they may "suffer in silence," hoping their physician will some how miraculously pick up on their problem and treat it. A more realistic approach might be to tell your doctor, "I realize that this sounds a little odd and it embarrasses me to tell you this, but my tongue tingles." You must also form the habit of being honest with yourself. If you have not been taking your medication, following your diet, or making the effort to exercise, admit it to yourself. Don't blame anything on anyone else. It does not help. Start again. Many MVP patients tend to fool themselves in a number of ways. Becoming progressively worse, they may convince themselves that the entire world needs to sleep 18 hours a day. A few of my patients are in rather unpleasant job situations and would really like to quit and find something else. They should just say so and do so, rather than blame their MVP for their inability to do a certain job or keep certain commitments.

Changing Physicians

There are times when I believe that it is appropriate to seek the care of a different physician. If your physician is openly hostile to you, examine honestly whether you have been guilty of any of the "ways to turn off your physician." If you haven't, I recommend that you sit down and discuss your concerns with your physician. I say this knowing full well that you probably will not do it. Why? Because confrontation is unpleasant to most of us and MVP patients are generally not very assertive individuals.(One of the most enjoyable things I do is assertiveness training for MVP patients.) If assertiveness classes are not available to you, it would be wise to read the chapter on positive-mental attitude, and some selections from the suggested reading. Try this with your physician. It might accomplish a couple of things. First you might be able to work out a mutually satisfactory relationship with your physician, which could save you a great deal of time and money. Going to a new physician usually means a repeat of costly diagnostic procedures, as well as a series of visits required for him or her to become familiar with your case. Time is money. Second, if you can sit down and discuss things with your physician, you will have a positive experience under your belt. There is very little that encourages assertive behavior like successful experiences. It seems that the greater the difficulty of the experience that you undertake and succeed, the more confidence you gain in your ability to face and solve your own problems.

I would include in "reasons to seek a new physician" those rare instances when your physician might recommend some treatment or diagnostic procedure that is rather extreme. An example of this is the electric shock treatment recommended for the young woman suffering "blues and fatigue." Clearly, she would have been better served to have sought a second opinion. Another time might be when a physician recommends a cardiac catheterization to a young female with no family history of coronary disease. (Recall that a cardiac catheterization is the insertion of a catheter directly into the heart to inject dye and visualize the heart and blood vessels.) Cardiac catheterization is a very well-accepted, relatively safe, and very valuable procedure for cardiac patients. It is invaluable in determining the need for open heart surgery, and if you happen to have one of the very rare cases of MVP, that requires valve replacement, this might be appropriate. But it is not necessary for the average patient with MVP. Another time when catheterization might be needed is if you have one of the really dangerous types of heart rhythms or irregularities. Once again, this is very rare. In patients with chest pain, it is necessary to rule out coronary artery disease. Thus, a cardiac catheterization might be indicated for a patient whose primary complaint is chest pain. It usually is not done, however, unless your family history indicates a problem or you are over the age of 40. If a catheterization is recommended for you, I might suggest getting a second opinion from a physician from a different group or even a different hospital. (It does not count to get an opinion from your doctor's partner and best friend).

What about the physician who recommends the psychiatrist? Should he or she be dumped? Not necessarily. Most of us can benefit from some insight into our own thinking and behavior. I consider myself relatively healthy emotionally, yet my shelves are full of self-help books (I refer to them as "rah-rah" books). I believe that we can all benefit from positive thinking. The MVPer's can surely benefit from guidance into better ways to relate to their rather unusual symptoms. They can also benefit from tips on how to avoid the pitfalls the MVP patient commonly encounters, such as the tendency to dwell on the condition to an excess. (Remember somatic preoccupation?) Learning ways to manage marriage and family relationships as well as those at work can be invaluable to patients with MVP. At the center where I work we have the services of an excellent clinical psychologist who does numerous psychological tests and conducts group and individual sessions for patients with similar problems, such as panic disorder, fatigue, and lack of assertiveness as well as sessions for families of prolapse patients. These have probably proven to be some of the most valuable services of the center, and our patients quickly realize we are not providing these services because we feel they are crazy, but rather because all of us can benefit from better attitudes toward our health.

I have mentioned that there are some MVP patients who, like many people without prolapse, are neurotic. These patients can surely benefit from psychiatric guidance. Extreme care should be used in selecting a psychiatrist. Many psychiatrists know as little about MVP as other specialists. Some immediately prescribe antidepressant medication, which can sometimes complicate the already delicate autonomic nervous system balance. Great care should be exercised to find a psychiatrist who will coordinate his or her efforts with those of your other physicians in prescribing medication. Psychiatrists and clinical psychologists have a great deal of experience in dealing with panic attack and agoraphobia (abnormal fear of open spaces or crowds), which is common in MVP patients. A good psychiatrist or psychologist could be a great deal of help in finding ways to overcome these tendencies. To choose a psychiatrist or psychologist, schedule an interview. Yes, you sit down and interview the professional. Certainly organize your thoughts before you go in and be prepared to ask questions (taking a few notes with you is fine — just not pages and pages). A few sensible questions might be "Have you treated very many patients with MVP?", "What types of problems do you commonly find in these group of patients?," "How much will it cost?", and "Is medication usually needed?." Remember that this is an exercise in assertive living that is absolutely vital to your future. Try it!

Finding a Doctor

Let us assume that you do not already have a physician, or that you want to change physicians. How do you go about finding a doctor with whom you feel comfortable? Do you choose a family practitioner, an internist, or a cardiologist?

Finding a doctor may be very difficult if you happen to live in an area where MVP has not received much attention. I would begin by asking friends. This may or may not work for you. Some people respond well to physicians who have a very authoritative manner; others prefer the very warm friendly manner. Whatever you are comfortable with is fine. I do strongly suggest that you sit down with him or her initially and discuss your problems. You could provide a very limited history of your previous experience with physicians. A warning here: physicians tend to stick together as a profession. If you go into a lengthy discussion of all the problems you have had with a number of previous physicians, I can assure you that this one will form the opinion that you are a "doctor shopper" and are difficult to deal with. It might be even better to put all of your previous experience behind you and start with a clean slate.

I do not have any strong feelings about the type of physicians who should care for the MVP patient. I work with a large number of young women and men in training for family practice. Their training is excellent. Internists also have a great deal of training in the area of cardiovascular diseases. Cardiologists, of course, are the most familiar with these conditions. But cardiologists can be expensive. The average MVP patient probably doesn't need the expertise of a cardiologist, although a rare few do need it. Fortunately, I have the benefit of the services of excellent cardiologists and a large group of physicians of all specialties to whom I can refer patients. If you would feel better under the care of a cardiologist then that's fine. But I really do not believe this is necessary in most cases. A far more important criterion for the selection of a physician would be a compassionate and patient manner.

Once you reach the point of stabilization, you will need no more health care than the average person, which may mean regular physical examinations and visits for colds and flu. I do not believe that because you have MVP, you must be seen on a regular basis. Some MVP patients must, however, be under the care of physician to regulate medication while they are being stabilized. I see new patients after six weeks and again at three months.

About Your Insurance

Most people in this day and age have insurance. It is hard to imagine how a person could handle unexpected medical expenses without it. There are many different insurance companies and each has many types of plans. All of us should be aware of what kinds of medical expenses our insurance coverage will take care of and which kinds of it will not. Both fortunately and unfortunately for all of us, there has been an explosion of medical technology in the last decade. We are now able to take care of babies who would not have survived only a few years ago. We are able to diagnose and treat problems that were not even recognized previously. Some of the elderly and the terminally ill can be maintained almost indefinitely. Many of these advances are wonderful, but all are expensive. Health care can take a large portion of every dollar we earn. Far too many people believe that because insurance covers a certain type of treatment, the treatment is free. Wrong! We all pay for every diagnostic test in one way or the other. Until just a short time ago, if a person was admitted to the hospital for a work-up, any number of tests were done routinely. Some were not essential, just "nice to have." Much of this testing was done in response to the increasing tendency to bring malpractice suits against physicians. Out of self-defense doctors left no stone unturned when diagnosing or treating any patient. We simply cannot afford to continue this practice. My advice regarding insurance is simple — have it! Know what your insurance covers and what items you will have to pay for. If you need diagnostic procedures, see whether they can be done on an outpatient basis (many insurance carriers will waive the deductible fee if you have a procedure done as an outpatient).

Carefully monitor all diagnostic procedures that you undergo and watch for duplicate charges and charges for procedures that were not performed. Do this even if the bill is to be covered by an insurance carrier. Until just a few years ago, MVP was not recognized as a health problem. In the last few years there has been an explosion of requests for coverage of diagnostic procedures and hospitalizations, as well as other expenses, due to MVP. Some insurance companies still do not recognize MVP as a legitimate diagnosis. Be sure you check out your coverage, and be very conservative with its use.

Is there a lifetime limit to your coverage? A million dollars or a half million sounds like a fantastic amount of insurance coverage and is frequently set as a limit for a lifetime. True, the average person never uses this much, and you are not likely to need any more than average. But let's assume that yours is family coverage and you are unlucky enough to have a major automobile accident, involving a couple members of your family, requiring intensive care for several weeks and extensive long-term follow-up. There goes your lifetime allotment, and what will you do now? Although this rarely happens, I have seen patients who have to sell their homes and other assets because they have hospital bills that are no longer covered by insurance, but they are too young for Medicare. One of my favorite patients (not an MVP patient) recently underwent a successful heart transplant. As you can imagine, the cost was very high.

Above all, remember, that insurance or no insurance, you are responsible for taking good care of your health. It is nice to have good insurance coverage, but it is better to have good health and not need it.

Summing Up

In summary, the MVP patient needs the support and care of an understanding and knowledgeable physician. Sometimes, however, the nature of MVP symptoms can place a strain on that relationship by the chronic nature of the condition, as well as the lack of knowledge about the symptomatology. Every effort should be made to find the support of the right physician. You should be considerate of his or her time and frustrations regarding your care. However, if your best honest efforts to establish a good workable relationship fail, you must seek the care of someone else. Above all, remember that you are the consumer of health care. You pay for it and you have the right to expect compassionate care. Get what you pay for and cover yourself with adequate insurance, so that you will be able to pay. Again, the relationship between patient and physician is very important. Some of this relationship is dependent on the knowledge and personality of the physician; some, however, is in your hands.

4 The Role of Exercise in the Management of MVP

I recently read that there are four topics of great interest to all Americans today: diets, exercise, sex, and money. This particular article advised that anything of value you want to convey to the public, should be approached in terms of one of these topics. We would probably all agree that fitness, or exercise, has been a very hot topic for several years now. Have you walked into a bookstore recently? There are literally dozens, perhaps hundreds, of books about fitness. Jogging is now epidemic in our society. Fitness centers are springing up on every corner, and there are stores that specialize only in exercise clothing. For the most part, I believe, this is a healthy trend. Statistics show that there is beginning to be a decline in the death rate from stroke and from heart attack. That is great, although it would be a mistake to say that this can be entirely attributed to the fitness boom. We Americans are also more interested in healthful eating than we used to be. There seem to be blood pressure screening centers on every corner and in every shopping center to detect hypertension, and medical care is improved with regard to treatment of cardiovascular problems. All of these trends tend to give you the message that your health is in your hands, that you are responsible for taking care of yourself. This is especially true for exercise. No one can make you exercise. We can only make recommenaations that are proven and safe. The rest is up to you. As a patient with MVP, you are probably beginning this chapter with a healthy dose of doubt, saying to yourself, "How can she expect me to exercise when I barely have enough energy to get out of bed in the morning, and some days not even that?" Be patient. I'll get to the specifics in a few minutes.

It is well known that patients with MVP perform poorly on exercise tests and have a very poor exercise tolerance. Almost all of my patients undergo a specialized form of exercise testing called the metabolic stress test (Figure 4-1). Uniformly, patients with MVP respond with much poorer results than even the typical out-of-shape American (Figure 4-2). The exact reasons for this are not clear. Many authorities believe that the faulty regulation of the autonomic nervous system is to blame and results in the inappropriate failure to dilate blood vessels in the arms and legs, resulting in the build-up of certain chemicals, such as lactic acid. Lactic acid results in fatigue that limits performance. Others believe that the fear that results

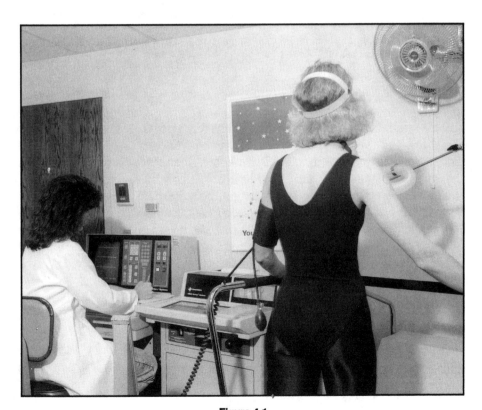

Figure 4-1

Patient Name: Jane Doe   Date: 4-27-87   ID#: 123456

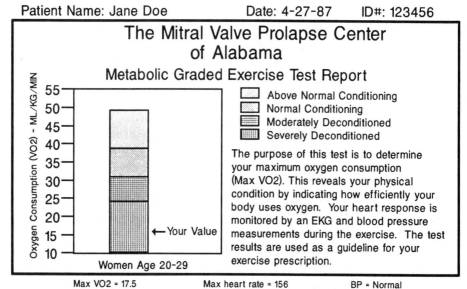

Max VO2 = 17.5   Max heart rate = 156   BP = Normal

According to the Metabolic GXT you are in very poor physical condition.
An organized exercise program is what you need to help you feel better, increase
your energy level, and help lower your blood pressure and heart rate.
You may want to contact the Center to receive information about exercise programs.

Figure 4-2

from the syndrome makes people do fewer and fewer activities until deconditioning
takes over. The symptoms of deconditioning are very similar to, and sometimes
impossible to distinguish from, MVP syndrome. Shortness of breath on mild exertion, inappropriate tachycardia (rapid heartbeat), the tendency for the blood pressure to fall upon standing, and markedly diminished exercise capacity are some of
the symptoms. I must admit that I have seen MVP patients who have been inactive
so long, that it was impossible to tell where the deconditioning left off and the
MVP syndrome began. Both deconditioning and MVP syndrome are vicious
cycles. Our aim is to break the cycle with very carefully chosen programs to reverse
the effects of deconditioning and stabilize the MVP syndrome.

Many physicians have stopped testing young females with MVP on the standard
exercise test because of the frequency of the abnormal results I've been describing and
because the meaning of these unusual results is not clear. However, I believe that exercise testing can be very valuable in a number of situations. First, in the patient with a
family history of heart disease, or in older females or in males, the test is needed to
rule out the possibility of more serious heart disease. Also a metabolic stress test
helps to establish your starting point for a program of reconditioning and rules out
any serious condition that may stand in the way of your progress. If exercise testing

is not available to you in your area, it is still a good idea to be checked out by your physician and to get the go-ahead before you begin any exercise program.

I was directing a program of cardiac rehabilitation a few years ago and quickly learned that it was useless to advise any patients of mine to "get some exercise." I had to be very specific with my recommendations and follow-up to make sure that I was understood. That's what I will do with you. I will tell you how to begin, what to do, how much to do, and how often.

Let's review for a moment some well-documented and well-accepted benefits of regular exercise:

- Cardiovascular fitness
- Improved Energy Levels
- Better Digestion
- Weight Control
- Improved Self-Image
- Relaxation

In general, regular exercise results in more energy, greater ability to handle stress, fewer physical complaints, less depression and anxiety, better digestion, less constipation, weight control, stronger bones that are less likely to break with age, better sleep, slowing of the aging process, better concentration, fewer aches and pains including back ache, and so on. This almost sounds like the old snake-oil salesman, promising miracle cures. But remember, anyone, anytime, at any age can benefit from regular exercise that is appropriately chosen for his or her particular limitations and situation. Every benefit mentioned would be appreciated by the prolapse patient, yet it is difficult to convince patients to exercise regularly, especially the person with the zero energy level. It is difficult for an MVP patient to make a commitment to exercise for a long enough period of time to appreciate the benefits. But if patients can be guided and motivated to make these commitments, they are greatly rewarded and see and feel the difference it makes in their lives.

Fitness

Although in the laboratory we have a very sophisticated method for determining your fitness level, there is no simple definition of fitness. For the purposes of this text, I will define *fitness* as the ability to perform the activities of daily living, both work and play, with vigor and without undue fatigue. Fitness has several important components, and it is inappropriate to concentrate solely on one or two of the components and neglect the others. Generally, fitness includes flexibility, strength, cardiovascular fitness (heart and lungs), muscular endurance, and weight as a measure of body composition. We will cover each component separately.

Flexibility is the ability to use the joints through the full range of movement.

Flexibility is required to move freely. Some people are naturally less flexible than others. Flexible joints are much less prone to injury than stiff, out-of-shape joints. As mentioned earlier, people with MVP frequently have very flexible joints. So flexible, in fact, that the flexibility itself may make them prone to injuries, even more than those people with very inflexible joints. For you it will be important to remain flexible, yet to avoid injury in exercising by choosing the right activity and using adequate safety precautions. To build or maintain flexibility, it is necessary to use specific stretching exercises, such as those listed later in this chapter. Stretching should be done slowly and should never produce pain. Researchers believe that as many as 80 percent of all back problems may be from weak, inflexible, muscle groups that support, or fail to support, the back.

The second major component of fitness is cardiovascular fitness. The heart and lungs are usually strong enough to circulate well-oxygenated blood to all the tissues of the body and to remove waste products of metabolism from the cells. In addition to the benefits of exercise to both heart and lungs, regular exercise also benefits the large muscles of the body. This benefit is perhaps as important as or more important than the effect of exercise on the heart muscle itself. Exercise allows all muscles to use oxygen more efficiently, thereby requiring less work from the heart and lungs. Without proper training, all muscles may lose some of their ability to function. "What you don't use, you lose" really applies here. Poor fitness can be very clearly seen in the older individuals who are seen in cardiac rehabilitation programs following heart attack or by-pass surgery. Many of these individuals have suffered rather severe damage to their hearts. Our studies indicate that rehabilitation programs do little to improve the heart muscle itself in these cases. But with regular exercise training, the muscles of their arms and legs begin to utilize oxygen more efficiently and effectively, and exercise capacity improves dramatically. Their bodies adapt to become more efficient and thus put less strain on their hearts. Many can return to work, and most report that they are able to improve their lifestyle dramatically.

Another component of fitness is of body composition. We have discovered that the old height and weight tables are not very helpful in determining how much a person should weigh. A football player, for example, may be less than six feet tall and weigh 240 pounds, yet only have a small percentage of body fat. A sedentary 35-year-old female may be within her ideal body weight range, by the charts, yet when examined more carefully, may show as much as 40 percent body fat. During childhood there is usually very little body fat. Although some children are overweight due to hereditary factors, they are also often underactive and can be helped by merely increasing their activity levels. Body fat, however, increases with age. The most dramatic increase in body fat occurs after the usual youthful activities, in college when the sedentary habits of adulthood begin.

Body fat can be estimated in several ways. The most common is the use of the skin-fold measurement, which employs special instruments to measure the thickness of the fat under the skin in certain areas of the body. These measures are totaled and used to estimate the percentage of body fat. The most complicated, yet the most accurate method of estimating the amount of fat within the body is immersion. This method utilizes an underwater scale to weigh a person who is submerged in water. Because muscle is so much more dense than fat, muscle weighs more. A lean person will, therefore, tend to be heavier in the water than a person with higher fat content, who tends to float higher and so weighs proportionately less under water.

When months or years of inactivity occur, the muscle of the body tends to become marbled with fat, much like a good steak. Inactive people may not notice a weight gain, but often remark that clothes just don't look the way they used to look, or that gravity is beginning to take a toll. The muscles of the body are actually shrinking from lack of use, and the weight consists of more and more fat and less and less muscle. Just as this process takes time to develop, it also takes time to reverse. If you want dramatic results, you may be sorely disappointed. To expect immediate results is unrealistic. The average (not ideal) female has about 25 to 28 percent of her total body weight in fat; 20 to 23 percent would be much better, and 18 to 20 percent would be ideal. The average male has 15 to 20 percent fat, with 15 to 18 percent being ideal. Athletes frequently have less than 10 percent fat. Although many of our prolapse patients tend to be tall and slender, because of months or years of limited physical activity, they tend to be proportionately fatter than their counterparts. When you begin a personal fitness program, I would strongly recommend that you get a measure of your percentage of body fat. At the very least, use the short-cut method outlined later in this chapter. Record the percentage and recheck the figure in six months or so. Yes, it really does take that long. It usually takes years to become really unfit, and it will take quite some time to reverse those changes. So don't look for short cuts. In the chapter on nutrition I talk about the few prolapse patients who want to lose weight. When you diet and don't exercise, half of the weight you lose will be muscle, not fat. When, or if, you gain the weight back, it will be 100 percent fat and you will be fatter than you were before you started. So don't start unless you are going to do it the right way. Above all, be patient.

Muscular endurance and cardiovascular fitness go hand in hand, but they are usually discussed separately. Muscle strength and endurance are required to do daily work and avoid fatigue. There is little doubt that muscle tone improves appearance. Good posture, for example, is sure to make anyone look better. Two people of exactly the same height and weight look dramatically different when one is very fit with good muscle tone and the other is not. The fit individual looks slimmer, because muscle is more dense than fat. Fit muscles also keep areas of the body such as the abdomen from protruding. There are a number of myths about strength and muscles. First and most common is that strong muscles are bulky and inflexible. The recommended strengthening exercises will not build bulky muscles. The second is that strength is good for men and not women. Good muscle fitness is important to both men and women and enhances both masculinity and femininity. In fact, heavy weight training is generally not recommended for the MVP patient.

One of the most important reasons to exercise is to avoid hypokinetic diseases, the diseases that are directly attributable to inactivity. A number of diseases, such as low back problems, and according to some authorities, diseases of the heart and blood vessels can be directly attributed to lack of physical activity. Less obvious are the diseases that result from constant stress on a daily basis. The fight or flight response that saved our forefathers was useful because they spent most of their days working, running, and climbing, to provide food for their families, blaze trails, or fight off enemies. Today this response occurs automatically in the body under stress, and results in the outpouring of certain hormones, such as adrenalin, into the blood stream. This can cause the heart to beat faster, digestion to slow, and blood vessels to tighten. This happens automatically in preparation for facing whatever the stress may be. Today, however, we do not forage for food or clear land to burn off these chemicals, and our bodies may remain for long periods of time in the "red alert" status. Ulcers, colitis, some headaches, and possibly hypertension and heart disease can be the result of prolonged stress that is not properly handled by the body. Because it can relieve stress exercise may be one of the most effective means for dealing with this problem. When you first begin to exercise, even the mild exercise I recommend, you may feel tired. Within a few weeks, however, if you persist, you will discover that this exercise is invigorating and something you look forward to in your daily life. I promise.

Before you begin any exercise program, as I have mentioned before, see your physician. When he or she has cleared you to start an exercise program, sit down with yourself and have a nice long chat. Make a commitment to exercise, starting today. No excuses. It won't be easy, especially on days when you feel pooped. Results won't happen overnight, and you will have good days and bad days. But within three to four weeks the results will start to show. You can begin to break your vicious cycle and reverse the process that has been getting you down for some time.

Exercise is not a panacea. It has many benefits, but it cannot cure all the physical and psychological problems of the world. It cannot, for example, cure or even prevent the common cold. And if incorrectly selected or improperly done, exercise may result in muscle strain, undue fatigue, and perhaps ankle or knee injuries. However, if the proper exercises are selected and you follow the exercise program with care, using certain safety rules, it can have dramatic effects on your general health and psychological well being. If you follow the guidelines in this chapter faithfully and be patient, good results will follow.

Principles of Conditioning

Three principles of physical conditioning are noteworthy at this point, the overload principle, the progression principle, and the specificity principle. The *overload principle* states that you must exert yourself more than you usually do to build fitness. Centuries ago the legendary Milo of Crotona was said to have developed strength by carrying a young calf on his shoulders each day. As the calf grew heavier and heavier, Milo was forced to lift more and more. The story illustrates the overload principle. You must do a little more than usual to gain fitness. At this point I must make a very unpopular statement. Housewives, even with small children, do not get enough activity from their daily routines to be considered fit. Women usually want to shoot me when I say that. They tell me that they run after their kids all day long, lift them, and lift groceries. Sorry, it is simply the wrong kind of activity and not to the proper intensity to achieve fitness. Housework usually puts less than 30 percent of the maximum work load on the body. In addition, it is intermittent. Fitness can be achieved only by stressing our bodies to a little more than 50 percent of maximum load and for a prolonged period of time, for example as 20 minutes of uninterrupted activity three or four times a week. Housework doesn't count; neither does golf, gardening, or shopping, for example. These activities are great for maintaining tone and for making you feel productive, and some are necessary for the function of a modern household, but they don't qualify as conditioning activities. Daily activities are cumulative, however, and are great to build into your lifestyle. Park your car at the far end of the parking lot each day and walk a little farther. Take the stairs instead of the elevator. Over months and years these activities will burn calories and keep you trim, but they can't be counted in your cardiovascular conditioning program.

Our bodies are not like machines that wear out with use. On the contrary, our bodies are designed to be active. They improve with use. Fitness cannot be stored. You cannot exercise like mad the first week of the month and remain fit the rest of the month. To attain fitness, you must exercise at least four times a week. To maintain fitness, at the lower levels of exercise that we recommend for our beginning MVP fitness program, exercising five to six times a week is preferable.

The *progression principle* states that you must start exercising slowly and increase gradually over a period of time. As fitness improves, gradually increase what you do until you reach an optimal amount of exercise for you. Many beginners choose the incorrect load of exercise, doing ether too much or too little. The old adage that if 20 minutes is good, 40 minutes must be better may not hold true for the MVP exerciser. Begin at a reasonably low level and progress very slowly. There is no hurry. It took a long time to become deconditioned, and you have the rest of your life to become fit.

The *specificity principle* suggests that to build specific components of fitness, you must select a specific type of exercise; for example, lifting weights improves strength but it does nothing for flexibility (remember I said I did not recommend weight training for the MVP patient). The best types of exercise build as many components of fitness as possible. For example, a daily walk improves cardiovascular fitness and improves body composition, but does very little for flexibility. If in addition to your daily walk, you carry "heavy hands" or some very light wrist weights, this routine can also build strength.

The Exercise Prescription

This chapter outlines a program that is safe and sensibly promotes all components of fitness. The *exercise prescription* is the term first used to describe a recommendation of exercise for cardiac patients. The prescription must be written, specifying the activity to be done, and the intensity and frequency with which the activity is to be performed. An example of a general exercise prescription might be:

Mitral Valve Prolapse

Aerobic Conditioning Program

30 minutes per day minimum

5 days per week minimum

Walking, swimming, bicycling

dancing, treadmill

The following is an example of an exercise prescription specifically for John Smith.

Name: John Smith

Date: 12-26-86

Walk two miles   in thirty minutes   five times weekly.
   (activity)   (intensity)   (frequency)

Aerobic Exercise

I will attempt to help you establish your own exercise prescription like the ones we develop for each patient I see. The type of exercise I am going to recommend is known as aerobic exercise. The term *aerobic* means living in air or utilizing oxygen.

Aerobic exercises are those activities that require increased amounts of oxygen for prolonged periods of time. When aerobic exercise, such as walking, bicycling, or swimming, is performed for 20 to 30 minutes at least three times a week, certain changes in the body occur that improve its capacity to utilize oxygen. Specifically, regular exercise improves the ability of the body to move air into and out of the lungs, increases the total volume of blood, and makes the tissues throughout the body better able to utilize oxygen efficiently. Aerobic exercise need not involve jogging and does not require excessive speed or athletic ability. I will stress over and over again the importance of prolonged, mild to moderate exercise. In other words, don't work harder, work longer. This is also known as the Frederickson LSD method (long, slow, distance).

Traditional rehabilitation programs, and most fitness programs, emphasize the concept of exercising in the target zone. You have probably heard of the formula 70 to 80 percent of predicted maximum heart rate for 20 minutes three times a week. Maximum heart rate is defined by subtracting your age from 220. For example, for a 22-year-old prolapse patient, 220 minus 22 is 198; 70 to 80 percent of 198 is 138 to 158, which defines the target zone. This formula may work for you, if you happen to be one of those MVP patients with a normal heart rate. Most of my patients, however, have rather inappropriate responses to exercise, and many have rather fast heart rates, even at rest. Heart rate responses to exercise may also be inappropriately high when deconditioning occurs. For these reasons, I have found that heart rate alone is a very poor guideline for exercise in the MVP patient. Elevated heart rate alone is not enough to produce fitness. If this were the case, some of my patients who walk around for several hours every day with heart rates in the 130 to 150 range, would be world class athletes. Remember that to achieve fitness you must increase the activity level to more than normal and sustain that activity for several minutes, several times a week. Another way that is frequently used in cardiac rehabilitation programs to guide exercise intensity is a scale that indicates "perceived level of exertion." For a given activity this scale indicates the level of exertion that the patients believe they are experiencing — for example, mild, moderate, or severe. This scale, the Borg scale, is useful, but it is not completely appropriate for MVP patients. When deconditioning occurs, MVP patients may feel extreme exertion with only small amounts of activity. If such a person were advised to pursue activities to a moderate amount of exertion, he or she might be able to perform only a few activities around the house, and would not achieve any meaningful degree of fitness. I often use a modified version of the Borg scale that can be quite useful with MVP patients (Figure 4-3).

I advise my patients to begin at lower levels of exertion and to increase the exertion weekly. I determine their fitness level based on a modified exercise test that I administer to each patient. I have patients tell me their perceived level of exertion on the exercise test so I can make an exact exercise prescription based on this level.

Rate of Perceived Exertion

6	
7	Very, very light
8	
9	Very light
10	
11	Fairly light
12	
13	Somewhat hard
14	
15	Hard
16	
17	Very hard
18	
19	Very, very hard

Figure 4-3

The Exercise Program

I usually recommend beginning a conditioning program by planning a specific time of the day to exercise. Many of my patients feel better in the afternoon and are more successful in following through with exercise at that time of the day. Others feel better in the morning and should plan to take advantage of that peak time.

I advise beginning the exercise period with about five minutes of gentle stretching exercise that also serves as a warm-up. Several examples are provided in "Exercises" at the end of this chapter. Stretching should be done slowly and should never produce pain. It should be followed by 5 to 15 minutes of very gentle aerobic activity such as walking, swimming, stationary bike (at low resistance), or treadmill walking. These activities should be performed very slowly at first so as not to result in excessive shortness of breath or undue fatigue. the exercise period should end with five minutes of gentle activity or cool down. The exercise session I've described may seem like very little activity, but often for a very out-of-condition patient it seems to be a lot of activity and is enough to produce fatigue. Because the intensity of the exercise is so low, it is necessary to perform the routine at least five days a week to achieve some level of fitness. After about two weeks at this low level, you will have progressed to the point that will allow you to begin a real conditioning program.

I have included a blank exercise prescription for your personalized program in "Exercises" at the end of this chapter. Remember to update your prescription every two to three weeks. If you have any problem determining your beginning level, ask your physician to recommend a level based on your exercise performance, or seek out the services of a qualified exercise physiologist. A blank personal exercise record is also included in the "Exercises" section. As with any other lifestyle change, be patient. Results take time, but the rewards are definitely worth it.

Type of Exercise

I believe that a good knowledge of exercise will help you to sort out which types of exercise programs or facilities may be helpful to you individually, and which types you would be well advised to stay away from. You must first learn some of the terminology.

Isometric Exercise

Isometric activities involve exercise that contracts muscles but does not move the joints and extremities. For example, pushing against an immovable object, such as a wall, is isometric exercise. Such exercises may increase the size of some muscles, but this type of exercise has no effect whatsoever on cardiovascular fitness. In fact, recent studies have shown that sudden blood pressure changes are associated with this type of activity, so isometric exercise may be an unwise choice for the MVP patient, who may already have problems with unstable blood pressure.

Isotonic or Isophasic Exercise

Isotonic, or *isophasic* exercises involve contraction of a muscle, and then movement of a joint, an extremity, or both during muscle contraction. Two classic examples of this are weight lifting and calisthenics. Another way to say this is that you use weight of some sort to resist contraction of the muscle, thus, putting a load on the muscle that results in increasing strength. This can be done on a weight machine or by using the weight of the body itself. Sit-ups and push-ups are good examples of this kind of exercise. Once again, this type of exercise does increase strength, but unless it's done for a prolonged period of time, for example, in an exercise class with prolonged calisthenics, it does not increase cardiovascular capacity. Weight training is very popular now, and many of my patients are very interested in participating in this activity. I will not tell you that it is absolutely contraindicated, but it is something that deserves a great deal of caution. The reason once again is not entirely understood, but the blood pressure changes associated with weight training, particularly upper extremity training, are frequently not very well tolerated by the MVP patient. A number of patients, however, have gone on the general conditioning program and after they have been stable for a number of months, have gradually begun a mild, weight-training program. If you are like most of the patients that I see, weight training is not the place to begin. Calisthenics requiring only minimal resistance, such as the single leg lift or a partial sit-up, may safely be used to add tone and strength to the body. There are also some very light arm or leg weights that may be added in time to increase muscle tone.

Isokinetic Exercise

A relatively new form of exercise is *isokinetic activity*. Nautilus and Universal weight equipment utilize this principle. For example, resistance is encountered in both lifting a bar and when returning the bar to its original position. Used alone, isokinetic exercise increases muscle strength. A variation of isokinetic exercise that is now gaining support utilizes a number of machines that, together, work all major muscle groups of the body. It is known as *circuit training*. You begin by doing up to 15 repetitions (lifts) in 30 seconds, followed by 30 seconds of rest before you start on the next machine. Some centers are requiring an additional minute or two of calisthenics between stations. This activity not only increases strength, but also achieves some cardiovascular fitness. Once again, I would not advise circuit training for the beginning exerciser or the MVP patient in general.

Anaerobic Exercise

Anaerobic means, simply, without oxygen. Anaerobic activities can be done only for very short periods of time, because they are so intense that the body is not able to supply oxygen at a fast enough rate to the tissues to maintain the activity for very long. Wind sprints would be an example of this type of activity. The person who runs the 100-yard dash as fast as possible is a wind sprinter. Often world class sprinters will not take a breath the entire 100 yards. Activities that are this intense can be sustained only for short periods, so they are not aerobic conditioning activities. Some studies have shown that world-class sprinters may not be very fit aerobically if they do not participate in anything other than sprinting events. How can this be? Once again we refer to the specificity of training. Sprinters work to develop those muscles and skills that allow them to sprint efficiently. Sometimes they do not concentrate enough time on general cardiovascular conditioning. This may also be true for some racquetball players, too. Racquetball can be a very strenuous sport requiring short bursts of intense speed and energy interspersed with periods of relatively little activity. A very good friend (a great racquetball player) and I went for a run. Actually this was more of a trot (I'm a slow jogger, but I can jog almost indefinitely). My friend pooped out after only ten minutes. She was not aerobically conditioned, although she was a superb racquetball player. I might add, however, that I do not have the speed or agility to keep up with her on the racquetball court for five minutes. Specificity of training!

Aerobic Exercise as an Aid to Weight Control

As I mentioned in Chapter 1, many prolapse patients are tall and slender. Although this is generally true, many patients are prone to weight problems due to inactivity or the effects of certain medications. I have also noticed that although many MVP patients are not overweight, many are overfat, by skin-fold measurements. This is because the lack of activity has produced smaller, weakened muscles that are loaded with fat. In the chapter on diet I cover methods of weight reduction, but I must stress at this point also that there is absolutely no sense in beginning a weight-control program using diet alone. It simply won't work. You can decide to spend the rest of your life hungry, or you can increase your activity and modify your eating habits somewhat. I assure you the latter is much less uncomfortable and results in the slim, well-conditioned muscles that we would all like to have.

There are numerous good books about weight control — almost all recommending exercise as an adjunct to diet. I have listed several in "Suggested Reading" that I have found particularly useful.

Let me share some information that has recently come out in several research studies. We Americans are chronic dieters. We are obsessed with slimness, and "the average American woman" diets most of any given year. When we diet (diet alone, not diet with exercise) on 1,000 calories a day or less, our bodies sense the situation, and being the wonderful creations that they are, adapt by slowing the metabolism to prevent starvation. This was probably useful hundreds of years ago when people had to hunt for food and might go several days between meals. The body probably requires about 1,500 calories a day to maintain balance. When it senses starvation and the metabolism slows in response, the body requires only about 1,000 calories to maintain balance. At this point weight loss slows dramatically. Many dieters give up if they have not reached their goal at this point and try to return to somewhat sensible eating habits of 1,200 to 1,500 calories a day to maintain their weight loss. But it doesn't work. On 1,200 to 1,500 calories a day, you will regain the weight quickly, because the slow metabolism persists long after the diet has been abandoned. Many experts say that lower metabolic rates can persist for as long as one year after the diet. This bit of information makes it clearer why so many people yo-yo dieting, gaining weight, and starting a new diet.

Another complication of extreme dieting is that the weight lost, is about 50 percent fat and 50 percent muscle. When you regain weight, however, it is 100 percent fat, so you become fatter than when you started. After several diets you can imagine the results. Let's look at Suzie Yo-Yo, the chronic dieter. She goes on the "Beautiful Burbank Diet", (500 calories a day), and she loses 10 pounds in two weeks. Doesn't that sound great? Not really. In the first place, it is physically impossible to burn away 10 pounds of fat in two weeks. Probably five pounds of the weight loss is fluid. Remember that I said that patients with mitral valve prolapse have a tendency to have a low blood volume to begin with. Further loss in fluid from dieting can really increase MVP symptoms. In addition, the first few glasses of water in the first few days of normal eating will replace that lost fluid. The remaining five pounds that is a true weight loss is half fat and half muscle. Therefore, when she regains the weight, as she probably will because she has been so deprived for so long and because her metabolism has been slowed, all of what she regains will be fat. You can see that after a few months and a half dozen fad diets, she will be in much worse shape than she was to begin with as far as body composition is concerned.

Suzie is by no means unique. She is like millions of women in this country. The truth is that there are no short cuts. The only way to maintain normal body metabolism while lowering your caloric intake is to exercise regularly. Exercise maintains your normal metabolism so that you burn calories. There is no other way. So quit damaging your body and begin today to establish good healthful eating and exercise habits. A healthy and fit body is able to metabolize calories better than an overfat, sluggish body. Thus, when you are fit, you are better able to handle the calories that you do take in, and an occasional splurge won't be as damaging to you as it would be to the overfat, underfit individual.

Enjoying Exercise

Any program that you begin for your health, or for weight control, or for your figure, but that you hate, will quickly be abandoned. You can easily find excuses not to exercise on any particular day. I once read a clever list of reasons why a person should not exercise, such as: it's too: hot, cold, wet, dry, early, late, and so forth. If you want to find an excuse, you can. To enjoy exercise you must first accept that there are benefits that you want from the program, such as weight control, control of fatigue, and cardiovascular fitness. This kind of motivation is important, but it is not enough. Many of us know that certain things are good for us, but that does not make us follow through. You must choose activities that you really enjoy, preferably activities that you can enjoy for the rest of your life. It would be unwise to choose gymnastics as your major aerobic activity, even though this is excellent for your cardiovascular system. Have you ever seen a 50-year-old on uneven parallel bars? A better choice might be a vigorous walking program. Finally, you must make a commitment to your program for at least eight weeks. Most dropouts do so in the first few days to two weeks of a program. If a person stays with a program for as long as eight weeks, the results begin to be apparent, and that person is more likely to stick with the program.

MVP and Lack of Self-Confidence

You may already accept that exercise is good for other people, but still secretly believe that it is not for you. You may have had an experience in the past that strengthened this feeling. Many MVP folks can remember, even in childhood, never being quite able to keep up with their peers during physical education classes. Over time many patients develop a poor self-image regarding their bodies and their physical abilities. In addition, they may be afraid of exercise and what it will do to their shortness of breath, chest pain, dizziness, and so on. They may also be embarrassed to exercise with anyone around in case they feel faint or "lose control." Past experiences may make them hesitant to undertake an exercise program. "Learned helplessness" is a term that describes the attitude of people who feel incompetent in a particular endeavor. Where exercise is involved, prolapse patients are particularly prone to this. Many have learned from their own bad experiences that their efforts will not be rewarding. Part of their hesitance is due to the emphasis that society places on performance (how fast you can run, etc.), rather than on participation. Starting at an early age, children learn which types of activities they can succeed at and which produce poor results, or in the case of MVP, those that cause symptoms; and they begin to avoid these activities. This carries over into adult life. Many adults are secretly afraid of physical activities because they have learned that they have problems, and they don't even want to try. If you feel this way, you're not alone. You too can develop self-confidence, and you can enjoy these activities.

The secret is to take one step at a time. Success breeds success. Right now just look at the beginning level of activity, which is very low. Don't think about what kinds of activities you are going to be doing a year from now. Most successful patients have started by walking very slowly for short distances, gradually increasing both the distance and the speed. "Gradually" is the key word for everyone, but especially the prolapse patient. After you have been cleared by your physician to begin a fitness program, begin to look around for an exercise opportunity that fits your needs. Of course, you can exercise for free. Many people, however, feel much more secure if they are in some sort of structured program. A program specifically designed for MVP patients is very rare. There are cardiac rehabilitation programs that offer supervision. You must be careful, however, that they use special criteria to evaluate your exercise and do not put you in a class with all the other cardiac rehabilitation patients. You simply must have your own set of rules. You might also feel better if you contract with friends. Exercising with a friend is a good way to keep you motivated and to provide security in case a problem should arise.

I will discuss the pros and cons of spas and health clubs later in this chapter. But the key word for success in any structured program is patience. Set your program to progress gradually. If you try to progress through a preset exercise program very rapidly, you will be setting yourself up to fail. Never, never set yourself up to fail. Set yourself up to win, and above all, do not be a yesbut. Open your mind. From this moment forward put your past experiences behind you where they belong. They are past. Start fresh. You can be successful and you can feel better. One of Frederickson's major laws is "I will not be a yesbut."

Although I deal mostly with young patients, I do have patients of all ages, both male and female. Older individuals are generally less willing to participate in any exercise program. Older Americans generally are less active with each passing year. Should they be? Need they be? Many older people experience what is called *acquired aging*. This is the process of declining physical function, due to physical inactivity, mental inactivity, or both. Inactivity of older people is frequently the result of overprotective families who advise them to "take it easy." They then suffer loss of function from their sedentary lifestyle. It is never too late to get fit. I have seen individuals in their 70's institute a safe and sensible exercise program, and they are often my most committed and enthusiastic participants. Remember that you need not be an athlete to be active. There is a delightful line from *Walden* by Thoreau: "The woods would be very silent if no birds sang except those that sang the best." I have that pinned to the bulletin board in our exercise laboratory. You don't have to be the best or set any records. Just participate, and do your best.

Set Realistic Goals and Timetables

Very few of the population are either physically or mentally able to become really great athletes. Likewise, very few are unable to perform at all. The vast majority of the population falls in the average range of physical activity. It is particularly important for the MVP patient to have his or her own goals. You must have your own goals. You can be judged only by your own standards. You have your own baseline, and you progress at your own pace. You should be judged for you and you alone. This is why you must not accept a canned exercise package. You may very well fall short at first and be sorely disappointed, not to mention sometimes being out quite a lot of money. As you establish your own fitness level now and set realistic goals, remember that your goals should be directed toward participation rather than competition.

The First Few Weeks are Tough

When you have seen your doctor and have been reassured that it is safe for you to exercise, perhaps uncomfortable but safe, you need to be aware of the reasons most MVP patients drop out of exercise programs, so you can avoid these pitfalls.

1. You may think, "What's the use?" You may believe that you are able to do so little that it will never get significantly better. In addition, you may experience even more fatigue or symptoms than usual. This is especially likely if you have had bad experiences in the past and lack selfconfidence, or if you expect too much too soon. You must be patient. Plan to progress only one step at a time. It takes time to learn that you can do it. You have made a commitment — stick to it.

2. When you begin to exercise, even at a low level, you can expect to feel muscle soreness and fatigue. Extreme pain is *not* to be expected. If this occurs, see your doctor. Slight soreness and muscle fatigue will disappear with regular exercise.

3. Your routine may seem like drudgery; especially if you have chosen an activity that you find you don't enjoy. Try another. Remember also that as an MVP patient you may enjoy a lift in mood and spirits as the exercise progresses. So when you find a program that is not too unpleasant, stick to it, altering it as needed.

4. You may not see results at first. Most programs advise that results take three to four weeks. This program is at such a low level that it may take six to eight weeks to see results. But they will come if you persist.

5. Don't cheat. You're only cheating yourself. If you do very little one day, don't get discouraged. Record it honestly, and the next day start fresh. Don't try to make up for yesterday by a double dose today. Start fresh every day, take one day at a time, and put slip-ups behind you.

Spas and Health Clubs

When you talk about health clubs and spas, you're talking about big business. There are excellent facilities, and there are operations that are very poor. Almost all are concerned with making money, as is every other business in our world today. Let me give you a few guidelines to help you get your money's worth. There are several types of programs on the market that you will need to evaluate. The most common is the "canned program." These are packaged as books, tapes, video tapes, and so forth. Some feature Hollywood personalities. (I am planning an exercise video for MVP patients myself). Some aren't bad. Others are downright awful. Most important is that there is nothing individualized about these programs. As an MVP patient you have specific needs. Before you invest in one of these programs, you should rent one or look at a friend's program to see if it would be something you could actually use. Look at the credentials of the person offering the product. Is he or she an expert? What does "expert" mean? Does he or she have training in exercise physiology or sports medicine? Just because the author is fit or has a beautiful body, does not establish that person as an expert. Does the program offer more than one component of fitness? Does it offer progressively more difficult routines as the person gains fitness, or is everyone assigned the same routine? Are there any no-no exercises included? (See "No-No's" Exercises section later in this chapter)

Before joining a health club or spa, check it out thoroughly. In general, club personnel may not be qualified either to diagnose or to treat health, fitness, weight, or figure problems. Some establishments make false promises or misleading claims about the benefits of their programs. Some programs are even potentially harmful to the MVP patient. There are, however, some reputable establishments that offer good facilities and provide group motivation. They provide a pleasant, relaxing, structured atmosphere where you can escape daily routines and participate in activities with other people.

There are some things you should consider before joining any club. As an MVPer you may not be able to participate at the level of many other beginning exercisers. This may be discouraging. If you find a good club that is staffed with an exercise physiologist or medical personnel, you may find that they are able to design a program especially for you. This is the approach of the Mitral Valve Prolapse Center. But if you join any program, don't be demoralized by others who are able to outdo you. Avoid, like the plague, passive machines, sauna-suits, body wraps, sauna baths, and rigorous classes. Passive machines that move, jiggle, roll, rub, mash, or vibrate various areas, promising to "break down fat cells" won't help you. Non-porous sauna suits that make you sweat are dangerous. They do not remove fat, but instead they dehydrate the tissues, which is especially bad for the prolapse patient. Body wraps that claim to remove six inches of fat in one treatment are hogwash! Sauna baths are very much in vogue now. I have to admit that I like them; but beware; they involve a very hot room — 140 - 190 degrees. Saunas can result in dehydration, and the MVP patient is especially intolerant of heat as are many people with cardiovascular conditions. I would advise against participation in any preplanned exercise program led by an adorable cutie in a skin-tight leotard and a painted-on smile with the "work 'em till they drop" mentality. I personally enjoy a structured exercise class, and I participate in some myself. But I choose a low-impact class (not a lot of bouncing) and one in which people can set their own pace. Remember, you are the boss. You are paying that leader's salary and must not be intimidated by "don't stop" orders. Allow no one to embarrass you, and work at your own pace.

Fitness Testing and Risk Factors

Check your heart disease risk by taking the tests in Table 4-1.

If you are in the low or average risk category, good for you. Regardless of how you rank, examine those areas that you can have some control over and begin today to modify them. For example, you have no control over your sex, age, or family history; but look at some of the other risk factors, such as smoking or too much body fat. What about number 10. Do you exercise regularly? Studies have shown that people with a very high risk dramatically shorten their life span and have all sorts of health problems along the way.

Table 4-1. Cardiovascular Risk Points

		1	2	3	4
1.	How old are you?	30 or less	31–40	41–55	55 +
2.	What is your sex?	Female		Male	
3.	Does your family have a history of heart disease?	none	grand-parent with HD	parent with HD	more than one with HD
4.	What is your blood pressure?	normal	a little high	high	very high
5.	Are you under stress?	less than normal	normal	above normal	quite normal
6.	Do you have other diseases?	no	ulcer	diabetes	both
7.	Are you too fat?	less than	normal	slightly above	very fat
8.	Do you smoke?	no	cigar or pipe	less than a pack a day	more than a pack a day
9.	Do you eat a high-fat diet?	no	slightly high in fat	above normal in fat	very high in fat
10.	Do you exercise regularly?	4–5 days a week or more	at least 3 days a week	less than 3 days a week	no

Total your points for the 10 questions. Use the scale to get an idea of your risk.

Rating Scale

15 or less = low risk   26–30 = high risk
16–25 = average risk   31 or more = very high risk

Cardiovascular Fitness

Before you can begin to improve your cardiovascular fitness, you have to know where you stand right now. Your physician may want to perform an exercise test on you, using a treadmill and a cardiac monitor, very sophisticated methods for establishing your cardiovascular fitness levels. Exercise testing, in general, is very wise if you have any of the several risk factors listed above or if you are over the age of 40 (35 if you are male). An exercise test is not without its drawbacks. It is usually quite expensive and your insurance may or may not cover this item. It is also well documented in the medical literature that stress tests, in general, seem to be less accurate for females than for males. In MVP patients in particular, the standardized tests that don't use the specialized metabolic measurements are difficult to evaluate, because the person may be so deconditioned or may feel such fatigue that he or she is unable to perform on the exercise test. A stress test uses cardiac monitoring during exercise on the moving belt of a treadmill or on a bicycle. The speed of the treadmill is gradually increased, as is the elevation (the steepness of the hill you are climbing), until you reach what is expected to be your maximum heart rate (remember your maximum heart rate is 220 minus your age). At this point, as well as during the test, your electrocardiogram is monitored to show any changes that would suggest disease in the arteries that supply your heart with blood. An exercise test is really an excellent screening test for heart disease, but I must say that it can be somewhat stressful, because it is frightening to think about exercise performance when you have been feeling fatigued for a prolonged period of time. A less elaborate evaluation is the one designed by Dr. Kenneth Cooper of Dallas, Texas to test Air Force personnel. The original test involves 1-1/2 miles of running, but obviously that's much too rigorous a program for the average MVP patient. A modification of this test is much more useful. In performing the 1-1/2 mile test, find a school track or some other measured distance if a track is not available. I advise a track because you can avoid the hazards of on the street, such as traffic and unfriendly dogs. Warm up by doing the basic stretching exercises shown in the "Exercises" section of this chapter. Begin walking at a slow pace, and steadily increase your pace to a comfortable level. If you are able to jog slowly some of the time, fine. If not, no problem. There is no pass or fail to any fitness test. We are merely determining where you should start with your conditioning program. Walk for the 1-1/2 miles if you are able. If not, do what you can. Record your distance. Don't be surprised or embarrassed if you fall short of 1-1/2 miles. Most of my patients do. It merely means that you have a lot of room for improvement. A few of my patients rate excellent on the cardiovascular fitness test, yet still have symptoms. If you are in this group, don't be discouraged. You may need to look more to the diet chapter for help.

Factors Affecting Your Tests

Motivation clearly plays a role in how your fitness test comes out. You may be willing to undergo a great deal of personal discomfort to "score" well on such a test. I think it is wonderful to get an honest appraisal of your abilities, but don't put yourself to bed for three days in order to score a little better on a test.

Strength

Muscle strength can best be tested in a laboratory with rather elaborate equipment, but once again you needn't have elaborate equipment to have some understanding of your strength level. Are you generally able to tolerate upper body or lower body activities better? Most women have very little strength in their upper bodies. Many men with MVP also have the same problem. Because weight training is not usually recommended for MVP patients, I have provided a few exercises that will increase your strength safely. Begin with only a few repetitions — five, for example — and gradually increase. *Caution*: If you have chronic back problems, be sure to get special clearance from your physician before performing any exercise.

Rating Your Flexibility

The ideal situation for evaluating flexibility is the clinical laboratory. There are, however, some simple and safe ways to evaluate your own flexibility at home. The same precautions apply to the stretching evaluation as apply to the other types of testing. Special precautions should be taken if you have a history of back problems. Above all, don't stretch anything so much that it hurts. Rate yourself as adequately flexible if you can perform all of the exercises easily, and poor in flexibility if you have difficulty with any of the exercises. *Note*: The special exercises provided later in this chapter can dramatically improve flexibility if you have problems in this area. Even if you rate your flexibility as adequate, I still recommend stretching daily to improve general tone and prevent problems in the future.

Tests For Body Composition

As previously discussed, although many prolapse patients are quite thin, many have weight problems, primarily due to the inactivity that frequently accompanies their symptoms. Many are also overfat, although not overweight. This simply means that there is too much fat on the body in relation to lean muscle mass. Unfortunately, many people have become obsessed with how much they weigh, rather than how fat they are. The terms overfat, obese, and overweight are often used interchangeably. They are not synonymous, however. *Overweight* simply means being heavier than other people of the same height and age. Weight/height tables are based on averages. They do not reflect amounts of fat. Lean body tissue, that is, muscle and bone weigh more than fat tissue and take up much less space. Another way to say this is that muscle and bone are more dense than fat. A fit person such as the football player mentioned previously can be overweight, yet not overfat. It is estimated that 25 percent of American children and 40 to 50 percent of adults may be too fat to be healthy. If you're *overfat*, you have more body fat than you should have for good health. Overfat for males is greater than 20 percent body fat. For females, it is greater than 25 percent body fat. *Obesity* is defined as more than 30 percent body fat for males and above 35 percent for females. The laboratory is again the place to get the most accurate estimate of body fat. However, some simple do-it-yourself tests can give a fairly accurate estimate of body fat, although the result certainly will not be as precise as laboratory methods. Many factors are involved in becoming overfat. Heredity and body build certainly play a role, as do factors in the home. In your home, food may be used to show love, soothe hurt feelings, celebrate (Thanksgiving, for example, is the socially acceptable binge), or to curb boredom. All of these factors play a role in being or becoming overfat, but none are insurmountable. With conscious attention to a sensible eating plan and regular exercise, you can achieve leanness. Perhaps the most insidious factor in the United States today, favoring overfatness, is what is termed *creeping obesity*. When people reach their adult years, their activity level drops dramatically. Look at your own past to high school or college. Physical activity was a way of life. We walked or ran to and from virtually every activity. Sports were also frequently a part of this time of our lives. When we arrived at adulthood and got that job, where we began sitting for large parts of the day, things began to change. Sports were less commonly practiced, and thus the number of calories needed to fuel the body for its day's activities dropped dramatically.

Weight gain does not come on suddenly. In fact, many people do not gain weight at all until they reach 35, but they are gaining fat. The muscles that were strong and healthy when we were teenagers, are used very little and begin to shrink. Muscle becomes "marbled" with fat, just like the muscles of the steer in a feed lot. To fatten the steer for slaughter, you feed him, but more important, you put him in a small space so that he cannot exercise. A person may reach 35 to 40 and feel proud that he or she has not put on any weight, not realizing that he or she has gained fat and lost muscles. If those wicked ways of too much food and too little exertion continue, believe me, the weight will come on.

The average American gains about two pounds a year. This amounts to 60 pounds between the ages of 25 and 55. Do you see why it's called "creeping obesity." You cannot be guaranteed a longer, healthier life by being lean, but lean people statistically have less risk of a shortened life than those who are overfat or obese. Those who are severely obese have a 70 percent higher than normal risk of a shortened live, and those who are moderately overfat have a 40 percent higher risk. Much has been written about the increased risks of diabetes, heart disease, high blood pressure, and strain on the weight-bearing joints of the hips and knees that come with weight gain. Even more important, most people look and feel their best, both physically and psychologically, when they are lean. Although I have said that height and weight tables alone are relatively inaccurate in determining body fat, I have included perhaps the most commonly used ones as a part of the overall body composition test (Table 4-2 and 4-3).

Skin-fold measurements to determine the percentage of body fat are best performed in the laboratory or by specially trained individuals. However an inexpensive pair of plastic calipers can be purchased for home use to make skin-fold measurements. To do a skin-fold measurement you must have a partner. You measure your partner, and your partner measures you. Be sure to follow the directions carefully to ensure accurate measurements. The calipers measure the thickness of the fat under the folds of skin. The test is relatively easy to do and is in no way uncomfortable. Use the illustrations that come with the calipers to help you follow the guidelines for making skin-fold measurements. Just three selected skin-fold measurements can provide a good estimate of the total amount of fat in the body.

If you are average according to the height and weight tests, but have good or very good levels of fatness according to the skin-fold test, it could be because of good muscle development, since muscles weigh more than fat. If, however, your body weight is in the normal range, but your body fat measurements indicate that percentage of body fat is high, you should keep this in mind when planning your dietary and exercise program.

In choosing your own individual exercise program, choose a variety of activities that you enjoy. Choose activities that do not depend on perfect weather. Few of us live in climates that don't have rain, snow, or extreme heat in the summer. A walk-jog program, for example, can be done on a school track when the weather is favorable and done inside on lousy days. You could also substitute other activities, such as stationary bicycles on less favorable days. Variety will be important to your program to avoid boredom. In the "Exercises" section I have given you sample programs to suggest where to begin. I include stretching and strengthening exercises in each exercise program, as I believe that we can all benefit from these activities.

When you have completed your fitness evaluation begin to form an exercise prescription choosing the activity as well as the intensity or duration and frequency

Table 4-2. Metropolitan Life Insurance Company
Weight and Height Table for Women

Height Feet Inches		Small Frame	Medium Frame	Large Frame
4	10	102–111	109–121	118–131
4	11	103–113	111–123	120–134
5	0	104–115	113–126	122–137
5	1	106–118	115–129	125–140
5	2	108–121	118–132	128–143
5	3	111–124	121–135	131–147
5	4	114–127	124–138	134–151
5	5	117–130	127–141	137–155
5	6	120–133	130–144	140–159
5	7	123–136	133–147	143–163
5	8	126–139	136–150	146–167
5	9	129–142	139–153	149–170
5	10	132–145	142–156	152–173
5	11	135–148	145–159	155–176
6	0	138–151	148–162	158–179

Weights at Ages 25-29 Based on Lowest Mortality. Weight in Pounds According to Frame (in indoor clothing, weighing 3 lbs., shoes with 1" heels).

Table 4-3. Metropolitan Life Insurance Company
Weight and Height Table for Men

Height Feet Inches		Small Frame	Medium Frame	Large Frame
5	2	128–134	131–141	138–150
5	3	130–136	133–143	140–153
5	4	132–138	135–145	142–156
5	5	134–140	137–148	144–160
5	6	136–142	139–151	146–164
5	7	138–145	142–154	149–168
5	8	140–148	145–157	152–172
5	9	142–151	148–160	155–176
5	10	144–154	151–163	158–180
5	11	146–157	154–166	161–184
6	0	149–160	157–170	164–188
6	1	152–164	160–174	168–192
6	2	155–168	164–178	172–197
6	3	158–173	167–182	176–202
6	4	162–176	171–187	181–207

Weights at Ages 25-29 Based on Lowest Mortality. Weight in Pounds According to Frame (in indoor clothing, weighing 3 lbs., shoes with 1″ heels).

with which you will perform it. If you happen to be a patient in a rehabilitation program, an exercise physiologist can help you formulate your exercise prescription. I can hear the yesbuts now. "Wait a minute. It's all I can do to get up and get dressed. I certainly can't think about walking, cycling, or skiing." You're right. You can't begin at this point.

Take a look at an example. Patsy Prolapse has been diagnosed for three years. Her symptoms include profound fatigue, chest pain, shortness of breath and migraine headaches. Patsy's fitness evaluation shows that although she is only 26 years old, she has the cardiovascular fitness of an 80-year-old. Never mind the whys and wherefores. She has to break the cycle and get back on her feet. She is profoundly deconditioned. We will begin by having her do simple stretching exercises each day — faithfully. In addition, she is told to do the listed calisthenics, which are mild, starting with only six repetitions and increasing very gradually. For cardiovascular fitness she is told to "walk one-half mile on flat ground (at a shopping center for example) in thirty minutes, six times a week". Although Patsy weighs only 135 pounds at 5 feet 6 inches, her skin-fold measurements calculate her to be 28 percent body fat. That is, her body composition shows that she is overfat, but not overweight. I do not recommend a reducing diet for a patient like Patsy. As her fitness improves, her muscles will regain their tone, and fat will take care of itself. At this point her fitness is the biggest priority for her.

Let's take another example. Cathy Click is a 32-year-old woman. She has taught aerobics classes for the past eight years. She is in excellent physical condition. She runs 15 miles a week and works out with Nautilus several times a week. Her symptoms include fatigue, palpitations (fluttering, heartbeats), and numbness of the extremities. Her blood pressure is quite low. Because she is active, she has never had a weight problem. But she has conditioned herself to reach for something sweet every time she feels fatigued. For her conditioning program I suggested that she back off just a little on the weight training, until the other factors are stabilized. She maintains her fitness by stretching, strengthening, and aerobic exercises. The main area that we will work on with her is her diet. Foods are discussed in more detail in the chapter on diet.

Mary Mitral is also quite deconditioned. As a 46-year-old female with shortness of breath and fatigue, she has been virtually incapacitated for the last four years. She has no flat area close to her home for walking. Therefore, I recommend the stationary bicycle, in addition to her stretching exercises and gentle calisthenics. She has started at very low levels, with very low resistance, and is gradually increasing as her fitness improves. Mary is also very overfat. She has approximately 30 pounds to lose. I recommend that she not count calories at this time, but rather avoid all sugar and caffeine and dramatically limit her fat intake. By increasing her physical activity and only moderately modifying her intake, she will probably lose weight very gradually. But even if she does not lose weight, she will be improving her body composition by increasing the amount of muscle and gradually decreasing the amount of fat. She will probably also lose inches and come out way ahead, without feeling much deprivation and without becoming dehydrated.

Now is the time to start planning your own reconditioning program. First, plan to do all of your stretching exercises, even if it is a particularly bad day for you and you are not feeling very well. Do them without fail. Next do a set of calisthenics (see "Exercises"). You may be able to do only one or two of each type of exercise when you begin. That's fine. Do them gently, and record how many you are able to do. Progress sensibly. You need never set a goal to do 500 modified push-ups. That's ridiculous. The purpose is to tone, firm, and strengthen your major muscle groups. If you can get to the point of doing 20 of each of the calisthenics eventually, wonderful. Firm, well-toned, muscles are great, but remember that aerobic conditioning is where the real payoff is for the MVP patient. That's what stabilizes the heart rate and blood pressure and gives the feelings of well being. It also reverses the deconditioning process and minimizes body fat. After the calisthenics plan to do at least 10 minutes of your chosen aerobic activity. If this does not seem to be enough and the sessions do not leave you overtired, then try a little bit more the next time. Remember, don't work harder, work longer (another Frederickson's Law). You might want to choose more than one aerobic activity — for example five minutes of stationary bicycling and five minutes of brisk walking. That's fine, but remember that aerobic exercise must be sustained for at least 10 minutes. Two five-minute sessions separated by time are not the same as one 10-minute sessions. When you have finished your 10-minutes plus of exercise, go to the "cool down" (see Exercises).

That's all there is to it. The first few weeks may seem difficult, and you may be very fatigued. But you must stick to it in order to feel the benefits. Progress to longer periods of aerobic activity when you can, but not too rapidly. Stay at one level for at least four or five days before progressing. Exercise sessions should be scheduled at least five times a week; six would be better, but not seven. Your body needs a day of rest, as does your spirit. But I promise you that you will soon begin to miss your exercise on your day off, and you may want to have a light session on that day also. Say, for example, a gentle stroll.

I won't pretend that this is going to be a snap — it's not. It may take every ounce of will that you can muster to stick to it, but I promise that if you make the effort and the commitment, the payoff will be great. Remember the old adage; What you don't use, you lose.

The MVP Exercises

The rest of this chapter provides exercises you can choose from in planning your daily exercise routine, as well as exercise records for tracking your progress (see pg. 112).

Warm-Up and Cool-Down Stretching Exercises

Perform these stretches before exercise as a warm-up and following aerobic exercise as a cool-down. Repeat each five times.

Neck Stretcher (to stretch muscles of the neck)

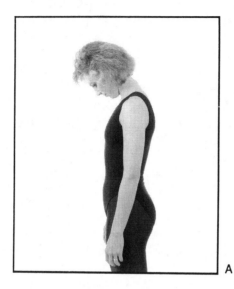

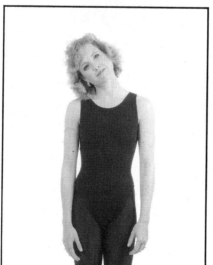

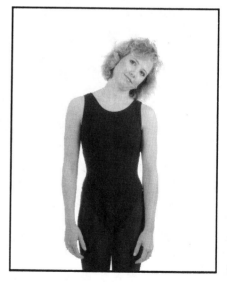

1. Bend head and neck forward, touching the chin to the chest (A). Hold for 5-15 seconds.

2. Tilt head to the right, trying to touch the right ear to the right shoulder. Do not lift the right shoulder (B). Hold the stretch.

3. Rotate the head to the left, trying to touch the left ear to the left shoulder (C). Do not lift the left shoulder. Hold the stretch.

A

B

C

Arm Stretcher (to stretch the muscles between the shoulders and under the arms)

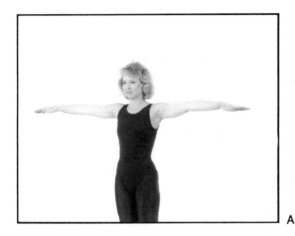

A

B

1. Extend both arms out to the sides at shoulder level (A).

2. Circle arms in 12-inch radius, 360 degrees (B). Do not allow your trunk to rotate. Repeat 4 times.

3. After you have drawn 5 circles, reach out with arms and fingers (C). Hold this stretch.

4. This exercise may be repeated several times during the day to relieve muscle tension.

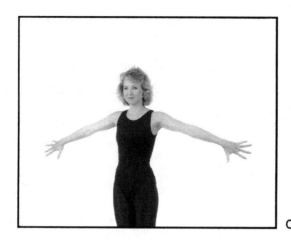

C

Chest Stretch

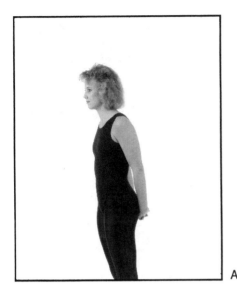

A

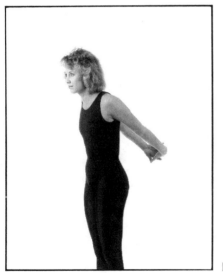

B

1. Bring both arms behind the body and clasp hands (A).
2. Raise clasped hands up to the point of stretch (B).

3. Return to the starting position.

4. Repeat 5 times.

Back and Leg Stretch

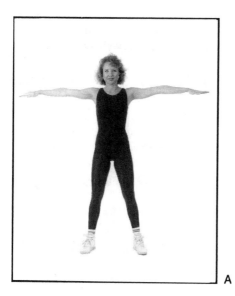

A

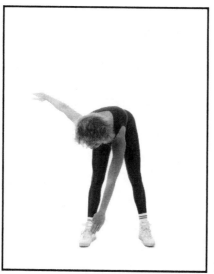

B

1. Stand with feet wide apart, arms outstretched at shoulder level (A).

2. Lean forward reaching toward the right toe with the left hand (B). Return to the starting position.

3. Reach for the left toe with the right hand. Return to the starting position.

4. Repeat steps 2 and 3 for a total of 10 times.

Pretzel Twist

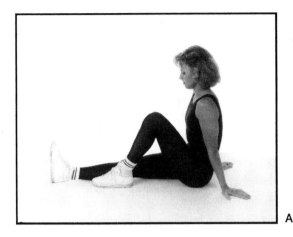

A

B

1. Sit on floor with your right leg extended in front of you and your left leg bent (A).

2. Hook your right arm behind your left knee. Turn to look over your left shoulder (B).

3. Hold for a count of 10.

4. Return to the starting position.

5. Repeat for the opposite side.

Fencer's Stretch

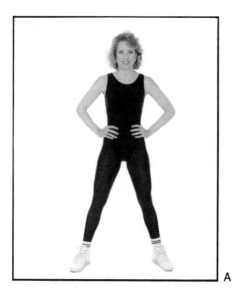

A

B

1. Stand with feet wide apart, hands on hips (A).

2. Bend the right knee and lean to the right side (B). (Right and left toes should be pointed straight front.)

3. Keep the left leg straight.

4. Hold for a count of ten.

5. Return to the starting position.

6. Repeat the same movements to the left side.

Rib Stretcher (to stretch the muscles under the arm and on the side of the upper trunk to relieve tension).

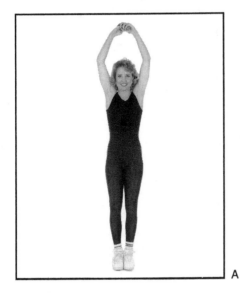

A

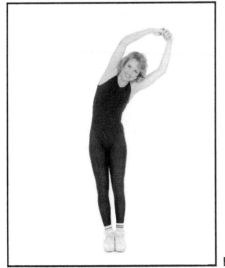

B

1. Lift your hands above the head. Clasp hands (A).

2. Use your left arm to pull your right arm to the left side (B). Hold the stretch for 10 seconds.

3. Use your right arm to pull your left arm to the right side. Hold the stretch for 10 seconds.

Trunk Twister (to stretch the muscles of the trunk).

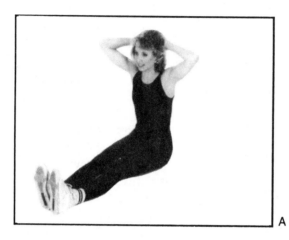

A

1. Sit on the floor with your back straight.

2. Clasp hands behind your neck.

3. Twist your trunk as far as possible, and look over your left shoulder (A). Hold the stretch for 10 seconds.

4. Repeat for the other side (B).

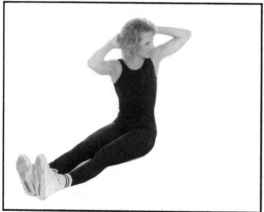

B

Hip Stretcher
(to stretch the hip flexor and lower back muscles)

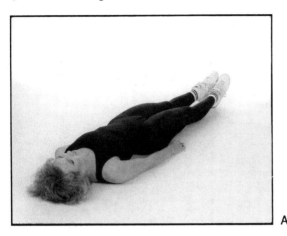

A

1. Lie on your back on the floor. Keep your back flat on the floor throughout the exercises (A).

2. Bring one leg to your chest, keeping the other leg on the floor (B). Hold this position for 10 seconds.

3. Repeat with the other leg

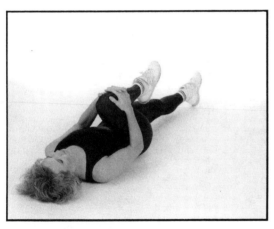

B

Low back stretcher (to stretch the muscles of the lower back)

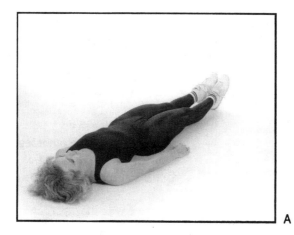

A

1. Lie on your back on the floor (A).

2. Bring both knees to your chest (B).

3. Use your arms to squeeze your knees to your chest.Hold this position for 10 seconds.

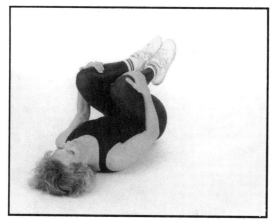

B

Inside-of-the-Thigh Stretch

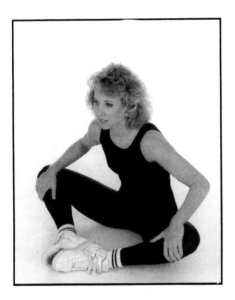

1. Sit on the floor with knees bent and soles of the feet touching. Grab your ankles and pull your heels close to your body.

2. Push gently down on your knees with your hands, and bend the upper body forward.

Calf Stretch

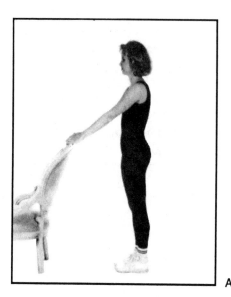

A

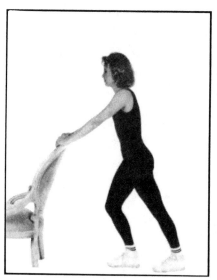

B

1. With both feet on the floor, stand facing a chair about 3 feet away (A).

2. Keeping the right foot forward and the left foot back, using your arms, lower the upper body slowly toward the chair (bend your arms.) Keep the left foot on the floor (B). Hold the stretch.

3. Repeat for the other side.

Hamstring and Back Stretch

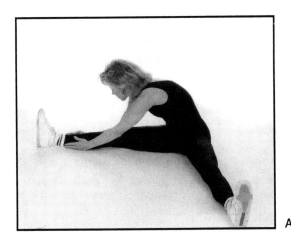

A

B

1. Sit on the floor with the legs extended as far as is comfortable.

2 Grab your right ankle with both hands and pull your head down (A). Hold for 15 seconds.

3. Repeat with left knee.

4. Spread the legs farther apart. Reach forward with both arms, and try to touch your head to the floor (B). Hold for 15 seconds.

Thigh Stretch

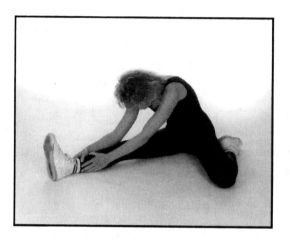

1. Sit on the floor with your right leg straight in front of you and your left leg bent to the left, your inside ankle touching the floor.

2. Try to pull your head to your right knee by grasping your ankle and pulling with your arms. Hold this position for 10 seconds.

3. Repeat after changing leg positions.

Arm Stretch

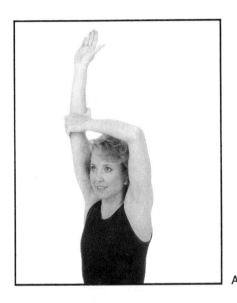

A

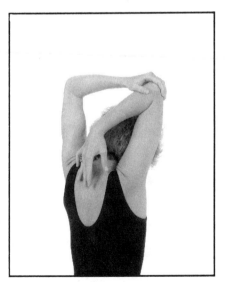

B

1. Reach over your head with your right arm. Bend your elbow and bring your right hand down to touch your back (A).

2. Using your left hand, press the right elbow back (B). Hold this position for 10 seconds.

3. Repeat with the left arm.

STRENGTH EXERCISES

The following exercises should be started with five repetitions and increased as tolerated.

Modified Push-up

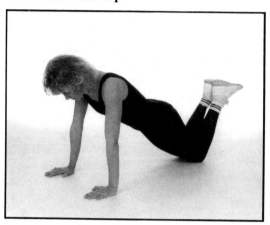

1. Bend at the knees, and support the body weight on hands and knees. Keep the body straight, and push up from this position. Return to starting position.

Modified Sit-up

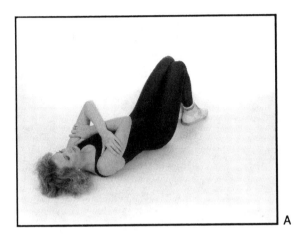

A

B

1. Lie on the floor with knees bent (A). This exercise is easier if someone stabilizes your feet or you lock them under a piece of furniture.

2. Raise your head and shoulders to the point that the shoulders are off the ground (B).

3. Slowly return to the floor.

4. Repeat 10 times, and progress as tolerated.

Knee-to-Nose Touch

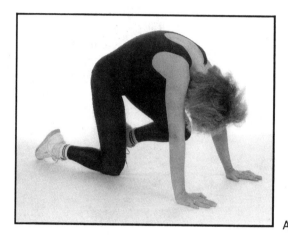

A

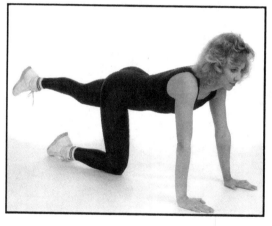

B

1. Kneel on hands and knees.

2. Lower your head between your arms.

3. Lift one leg and try to touch the knee to your nose (A).

4. Raise your head as you extend the leg out behind until it is straight and parallel to the floor (B). Do not lift the leg higher than parallel to the floor, and do not arch the back.

5. Return to the kneeling position.

6. Begin with 10 repetitions and increase as tolerated.

7. Repeat the series with the other leg.

Single Leg Lifts

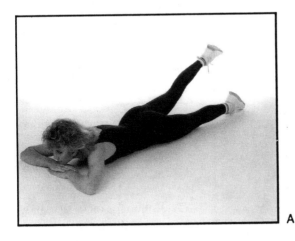

A

1. Lie on the floor on your stomach.

2. Slowly raise the right leg off the floor 8-12 inches. Repeat 10 times at first, and increase as tolerated.

3. Repeat the series with the left leg.

Side Leg Lift (Abduction)

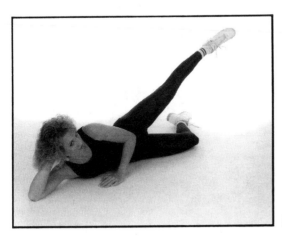

B

1. Lie on one side.

2. Raise the top leg as high as possible. (Lift the leg to the side, not in front of the body.)

3. Return to the starting position. Repeat 10 times and increase as tolerated.

4. Roll to the other side and repeat the series with the other leg.

Side Leg Lift (Adduction)

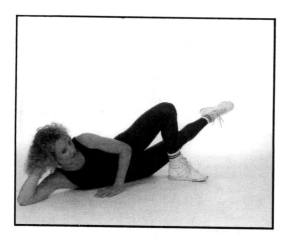

1. Lie on one side with your upper leg bent and in front of your lower leg.

2. Raise your lower leg toward the ceiling.

3. Return to starting position.

4. Repeat 10 times and increase as tolerated.

5. Roll to the other side and repeat the series.

Hip Strength

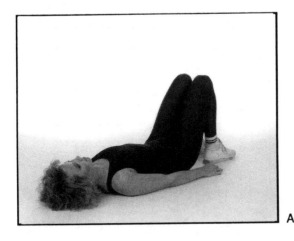

A

1. Lie on the floor with knees bent and hands to the sides (A).

2. Raise your hips off the floor 6-8 inches; squeezing the buttocks together (B).

3. Relax and return to the starting position.

4. Repeat 10 times and increase as tolerated.

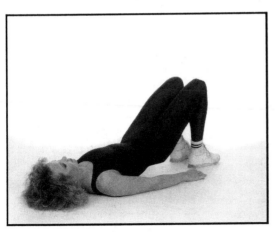

B

Back Strength

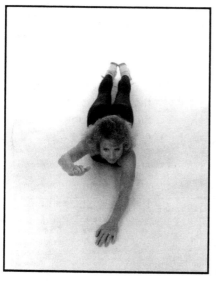

A

1. Lie on the stomach on the floor with arms stretched straight above the head.

2. Raise the right arm and hand 12 inches off the floor, hold this position for a few seconds, and return to the starting position. Repeat 5 times and increase as tolerated.

3. Repeat the series with the left arm.

Single Leg Lift

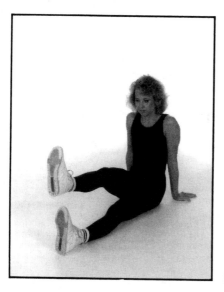

B

1. Sit on the floor with feet together and legs straight out in front.

2. Raise the right leg off the floor 8-10 inches, keeping the leg straight.

3. Repeat 10 times and increase as tolerated.

4. Repeat the series with the left leg.

Calf Strength

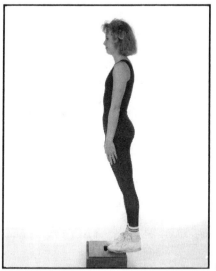

A

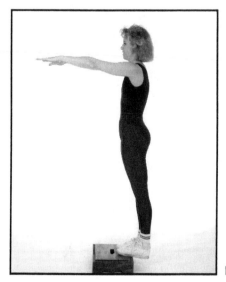

B

1. Stand with toes on a step or a large book; heels on the floor.

2. Slowly rise up on toes(A). Hold this position for a few seconds.

3. Extend arms, and return to the starting position (B).

4. Repeat 10 times and increase as tolerated.

Waist Whittler

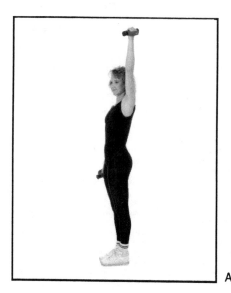

A

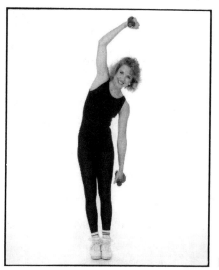

B

1. Use very light weights in each hand (2-4 pounds, no heavier) (A).

2. Raise your left hand straight above your head keeping your right hand by your side. Bend to the left side as far as comfortable (B). Hold for a few seconds and return to the starting position.

3. Raise your left hand and repeat step 2.

4. Alternate right and left for 5 repetitions. Increase as tolerated.

Firm Arms

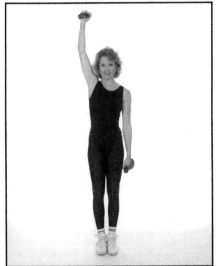

A

B

1. Using light weights, hold the right arm straight over the head (A).

2. Slowly lower the forearm to the back of the neck. (Be careful not to hit your head with the weight.)

3. Return to the starting position.

4. Raise the left arm and repeat steps 2 and 3 (B).

5. Repeat with each arm 5 times. Increase as tolerated.

Firm Upper Arms

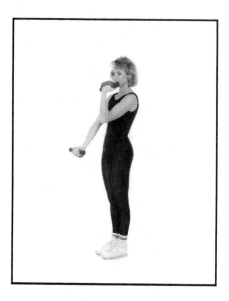

1. With light weights, keep both hands in front of the body, palms facing away from the body. Slowly bend the left elbow to bring the weight to the chest. Repeat 5 times. Increase as tolerated.

2. Repeat the series with the right arm.

Pelvic Tilt (great for low back pain)

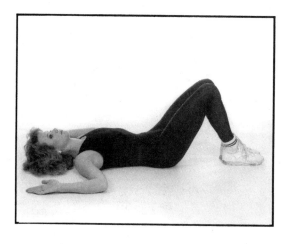

1. With knees bent, draw the abdominal muscles inward, causing the back to flatten against the floor and the pelvis to tilt forward.

2. Repeat 10 times and increase as tolerated.

EXERCISE "NO-NO'S"
(MVP patients should never do the following exercises.)

Extreme Arching of the Back

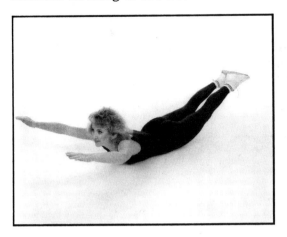 

Raising Both Legs at the Same Time

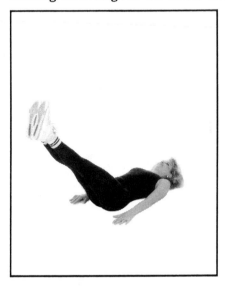 

Sit-ups with Straight Legs or Sit-ups with Arched Back

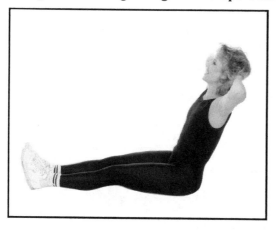 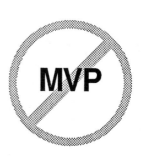

Deep Knee Bends

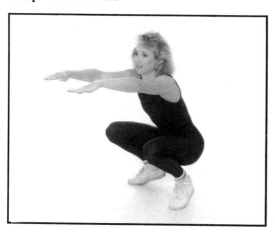 

Duck Walk

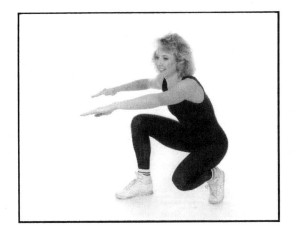 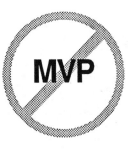

Alternate-Leg Deep Squats

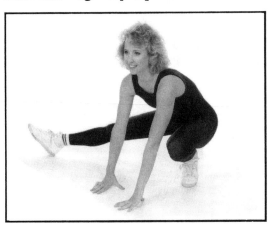 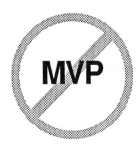

Heavy Weight Training

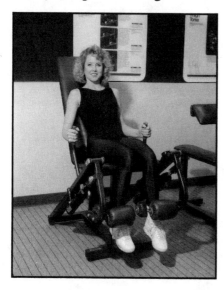
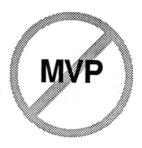

The use of heavy weights is contraindicated for the MVP patient. If you insist on weight training, use light weights and more repetitions.

Aerobic Workout

Benefits of Aerobic Exercise

- Cardiovascular Fitness
- Weight Control
- Improved Energy Levels

- Improved Self Image
- Aids Digestion
- Relaxation

Aerobic activity should be performed for 10 to 15 minutes and increased as tolerated to 30 minutes at least 5 times weekly. Recommended exercise includes walking, slow jogging, aerobic dance, swimming, stationary bike, climbing stairs, and treadmill exercise. Remember, the key is LSD (long, slow, distance). Working at low resistance for prolonged periods of time results in conditioning and improvement for the MVP patient.

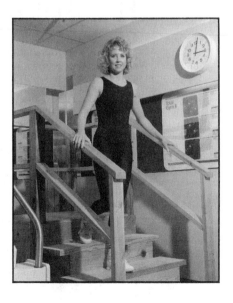

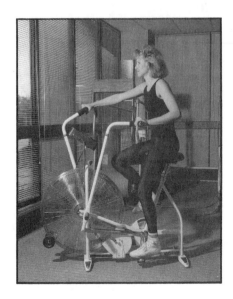

Weekly Excercise Record

	Mon	Tue	Wed	Thur	Fri	Sat	Sun
Activity							
Duration (Mins)							
Perceived Exertion							
Activity							
Duration (Mins)							
Perceived Exertion							
Activity							
Duration (Mins)							
Perceived Exertion							
Activity							
Duration (Mins)							
Perceived Exertion							

Notes _____

Date _____

5 The Role of Diet in the Management of MVP

I n our society almost everyone is diet conscious. But many MVP patients may want to skip this chapter. "I am tall and slender," they may say. "I don't need to diet." Some MVP patients do need to be on a special weight-reduction diet, but everyone with MVP needs to be on a high-energy diet. Food is fuel for the body. It makes sense that we should choose the highest-quality fuel in order to achieve the highest energy levels.

In any group of people you encounter at work or at a party, for example, you can probably pick out two or three individuals that you consider outstanding. Perhaps you would choose these outstanding individuals by appearance alone, but chances are you'd choose them partly because of their achievements and extremely high energy levels. You may be thinking, "Some people are born with high energy levels, and some are not; I just don't have high energy." That attitude will get you nowhere. Anyone is capable of improving his or her energy level with a properly balanced diet and exercise program.

You Are What You Eat

Good nutrition is the first step in a comprehensive program of total well-being for all of us, but especially for those with MVP and low energy levels. If you do not eat properly and have poor nutrition, it's almost impossible to undertake a program of physical conditioning or to achieve maximum performance, intellectually, psychologically, or spiritually. As I have mentioned before, the approach to MVP is one of balance, and one of the first steps is good nutrition.

MVP patients in our society tend to have certain predictable dietary shortcomings. Like deconditioning, poor nutrition is a vicious cycle. A patient may have a very poor energy level and not feel like preparing a meal, so he or she reaches for the simplest food source around, which is often loaded with fat, sugar, and salt. When we put this kind of fuel into the body, it makes sense that it is going to produce very little useful energy. The body requires good fuel to perform at maximum efficiency.

In addition to low energy making us seek out the fastest possible source of food, we also have a cultural problem to deal with. In our culture we "love" food, particularly sweets. Turn on any television set and you can see advertisements requesting that you reach for a Goo-Goo bar, or whatever, when you're feeling deficient in energy. We also use sweets for celebration. We use sweets for comfort when we feel depressed and as tranquilizers when we feel anxious. Caffeine provides another pitfall. Most people drink coffee, tea, or carbonated beverages, loaded with caffeine and often sugar. Caffeine is a drug, just like any other, and as mentioned previously, people with MVP are extremely sensitive to drugs.

When patients come to me for help with MVP, I request that they keep food diaries for the first three weeks. At the end of this time I sit down and review the food diaries with them, pointing out any pitfalls that I see in their nutritional status. The most common problems we see involve sugar, caffeine, salt, and fats. You may say "I don't have to worry about fat. I am already very slender." Remember, even if you're quite slim, you might be overfat. Also if you eat too many fatty foods, you usually limit the other more nutritious foods in the diet, such as the complex carbohydrates that are essential for high energy. Fats are slowly digested and do not tend to give you quick energy.

Caffeine

Before we outline a specific eating program, let's tackle the common problems one at a time, starting with caffeine. Caffeine is a stimulant. Remember, we mentioned that the autonomic nervous system is extremely sensitive to all drugs. The effect of caffeine is to give a sudden boost to the autonomic nervous system, followed by a plunge. Caffeine stimulates the release of adrenalin, which gives a boost that is then rapidly followed by a letdown. This sets the individual up for a "roller coaster" response of the autonomic nervous system, which is destabilizing. We have talked about equilibrium, or balance, being the key to controlling the symptoms of MVP syndrome. It therefore makes sense to remove anything that destabilizes the autonomic nervous system. If you are a coffee or tea drinker, substitute decaffeinated coffee and decaffeinated tea in your diet. If you have to drink a soft drink, drink the decaffeinated, sugar-free variety. But even those should be severely limited, for reasons we will cover later. (Remember, you chocoholics, that chocolate is also loaded with caffeine, sugar, and fat, virtually all of the problem substances you need to avoid.) Here is a list of caffeine sources:

Common Sources of Caffeine

Soft drinks
  Coca-Cola
  Mr. Pibb
  Mountain Dew
  Dr. Pepper
  Pepsi Cola
  RC Cola
  Shasta Cola
  Tab
  Mello Yello

Coffee
Tea
Cocoa
Chocolate milk
Chocolate, light and dark
Medications (see Chapter 6)

Let's discuss caffeine in more detail. In our society it is a socially acceptable drug, but it is a drug nevertheless. It also tends to be addicting, and many of my patients report that when they attempt to dramatically limit their caffeine intake, they experience severe headaches. For these and all patients, I advise that they taper off their caffeine intake by cutting their caffeine in half, substituting decaffeinated coffee or tea for the caffeinated variety for a week, then cut it in half again, and then cut it out completely. This seems to prevent the headache response. Cutting out caffeine is often difficult for that group of patients with prolapse who are subject to frequent severe headaches. If you are in that group, you may need to check with your doctor about reducing your caffeine intake because as you probably know, caffeine can often be used as a treatment for headaches. Caffeine acts on the blood vessels of the body and is often found in drugs used to treat migraines. However, if you can remove caffeine from your diet gradually, you will experience a great deal more energy and avoid its destabilizing effect on the autonomic nervous system.

Sugar

Next, let's talk about sugar. If I had to identify one substance that was absolutely poison to patients with MVP, it would probably have to be sugar. You may have seen the statistics indicating that at the turn of the century, the average American consumed less than five pounds of sugar per year, and now the average American consumes about 150 pounds of sugar per year. That figure is staggering.

Let's look at the effect of sugar on the autonomic nervous system. Have you ever eaten nice, warm donuts for breakfast and found that by 10:00 in the morning you're ravenously hungry? This hunger pattern is the effect of sugar. Your body responds to the sudden increase in the blood sugar level by pouring out insulin and adrenalin. As a result, the blood sugar level drops precipitously to a lower level than before the sugar intake. This results in the strong hunger feelings. Once again we are talking about a roller coaster effect on the autonomic nervous system. Pure sugar, and this includes honey, is a simple carbohydrate, which means it requires very little effort of the body to break it down and burn it. Complex carbohydrates, such as starches or even the more complex sugars found naturally in vegetables and fruits, require more time and energy to break down, thus giving the body a more uniform and stable outpouring of fuel.

Even if I have convinced you that sugar is bad for your health, you may still find it extremely difficult to break the sugar habit. There are several reasons for this. First, sugar is a highly addicting substance. We know that when sugar eaters try to limit sugar intake for several days, they become irritable, sometimes have difficulty sleeping, and often feel bad. This reflects a chemical withdrawal from sugar. If they persist, however, on about day ten they feel energized. I would challenge any of you to maintain food records like those in the "Dietary Records" section of this chapter, to see if you're consuming sugar on a regular basis. If you are, make a deal with yourself to avoid all sugar for two weeks. At the end of two weeks, see how you feel, whether you feel energized. Energized or not, go out and have a big candy bar and a soft drink. See how you feel then. Most MVP patients tell me that they experience a strong worsening of their symptoms when they do this. From that day forward, I never have to try to convince them of the negative effect of sugar on their bodies.

Cutting out sugar doesn't mean that from now on for the rest of your life you can never consume anything with sugar in it. That would be an unrealistic expectation. But you can dramatically limit your sugar intake to special occasions and small servings and keep it from being such a major part of your daily intake.

Fats

It would be prudent for all Americans to both decrease the total amount of fat in their diet and substitute a better form of fat, such as tub margarine, high in polyunsaturated fat, to reduce the risk of eventual heart disease. But I also have another reason for mentioning dietary fats. Women with MVP commonly experience symptoms of fibrocystic breast disease, that is, tenderness and swelling of the breasts prior to menstrual periods. For many women these symptoms are quite severe and uncomfortable. Amazingly, if you reduce dietary fat and caffeine, the symptoms almost totally disappear. You will find this will be another nice side effect of healthy eating.

It's very common in our culture to have an excess intake of fat. Even if you are blessed with a body that can handle it fairly well and you don't put on weight, you still need to limit your fat intake. Cholesterol and saturated fats are the subject of intense controversy in nutrition today. Vast numbers of scientific studies indicate that a diet rich in animal fats is strongly related to a high risk of dying young of heart disease, stroke, and even cancer. Most experts say that the evidence to support this is sufficiently convincing to warrant the recommendation of a diet lower in fats for all Americans. Heart disease, or atherosclerosis accounts for one half of the deaths in our nation. In this disease, material accumulates in the arteries, resulting in decreased flow. When the involved artery is supplying the heart muscle with blood and there is a decrease in flow (and therefore oxygen) beyond a critical level, a heart attack results.

The material that clogs arteries is cholesterol. After six months of age, you don't need to consume any cholesterol. Your body can manufacture sufficient cholesterol to meet its needs. The average American consumes 600 milligrams of cholesterol a day. Blood cholesterol levels begin to rise when the needs of the body are exceeded by intake. High blood cholesterol levels can result in deposits of cholesterol in the arteries.

The amount of cholesterol circulating in your body is influenced by the amount and type of fat in your diet. A diet rich in saturated fats tends to raise cholesterol. A diet rich in polyunsaturated and monounsaturated fats helps to lower levels of cholesterol. Saturated fats are generally animal fats such as lard, the fat on meats, butter, cheese, chocolate, egg yolk, palm oil, and solid fat shortening. Polyunsaturated fats are vegetable fats such as safflower oil, nuts, corn oil, fish oil, soft margarine, mayonnaise, and cottonseed oil.

That sounds simple enough, but it's a little more complicated than it sounds. Cholesterol is made up of three main types of substances, all called *lipoproteins*. These are high density lipoproteins (HDL), low density lipoproteins (LDL), and very low density lipoproteins (VLDL). You may notice these categories reported in test results if your doctor requests a test known as a *lipid profile*. The cholesterol number by itself is of little value. The ratio of the lipoproteins seems to be what's important, although, generally, the lower the cholesterol the better. HDL seems to be the good guy, acting as somewhat of a protection against atherosclerosis.

In our country there seems to be an elevation of cholesterol with age. This is not true in other parts of the world where heart disease is less common. The general rule applies that you should limit animal fat intake as much as possible. Substitute vegetable fat wherever possible, but in general dramatically lower fat intake altogether. As Figure 5-1 shows, fats should be limited to 30 percent of the daily caloric intake.

Many of my patients resist lowering fat intake, saying that they are simply too tired to cook the proper diet. They grab a hamburger (which is loaded with fat and salt) rather than taking the time to cook proper vegetables. Once again, your health is in your hands. You must take control of all of the factors in your life that you can. Nutrition can be the first step.

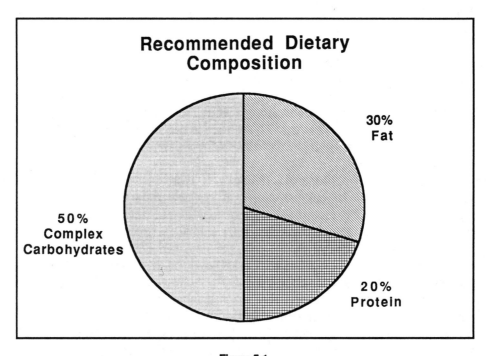

Figure 5-1

Fluids

MVP patients who are symptomatic because of a decrease in circulating blood volume have low blood pressure and a tendency to tire easily. These symptoms can be counteracted both by regular conditioning, which increases your circulating blood volume, and by maintaining a good intake of fluids--water, decaffeinated beverages, caffeine-free drinks, sugar-free soda, enriched fluids, and fruit juices. In general, most people do not get enough fluids in their diet. I recommend eight to ten glasses a day of fluids for MVP patients to maintain adequate blood volume and high energy levels.

Salt

Salt tends to hold fluid in circulation. Because many patients with prolapse do tend to be low in circulating blood volume, I usually do not dramatically limit their salt intake. I would, however, caution that if your blood pressure tends to run on the high side, you may need to dramatically limit salt intake.

Vitamins

Generally speaking, if you maintain a well-balanced diet with plenty of fruits and vegetables, limit the amount of fat in your diet, and eat plenty of whole-grain breads and cereals, you will take in enough vitamins and you won't need vitamin supplements. I don't think it's necessarily a bad idea to take a general vitamin supplement once a day, but we strongly discourage megadoses of any nutrient, as this can be dangerous. There is some evidence to suggest that because of our modern diet, consisting of foods that are largely refined, and because of the amount of stress in our culture (stress depletes the body's supply of magnesium), there is a need to add a small magnesium supplement to your diet. I believe that the evidence for this is inconclusive, but because a small supplement is relatively harmless and excess amounts of magnesium are excreted by the body, we often recommend that our patients take a magnesium supplement of about 500 mg a day. Magnesium is an essential nutrient required by every cell in the body. Stress diminishes the magnesium levels of the body, as do phosphates, which are present in a number of our foods. Soft drinks, for example, are loaded with phosphates which literally leech magnesium from the body. To our way of thinking, soft drinks are one of the primary reasons for our current cultural magnesium depletion. For this reason, I recommend that you limit your intake of soft drinks to no more than one a day. If you are able to do without them totally, that's even better.

Planning For Nutrition

Patients with prolapse often tend to have rather poor eating habits. For example, they often don't eat breakfast, eat a light lunch, and eat a large supper. Occasionally there is a patient who just doesn't feel like eating at all. Remember, food is the fuel for the body. It is impossible for the body to function properly without proper food. I am going to show you how to plan a well balanced diet that helps you achieve a nutritional balance for maximum energy. Establishing an eating plan like the one presented later in this chapter will help you get rid of excess weight (if you are overweight), slowly and safely, avoiding the diet roller coaster that you have perhaps experienced in the past. Now let's get to the specifics of planning your nutritional program.

I recommend that you get about half of your calories in any day from complex carbohydrates. Complex carbohydrates are found in fruits, vegetables, and grains. These foods are also loaded with vitamins, minerals, and fiber. They have a high water content, too, which makes you to feel full and helps to stabilize the blood volume problems that many prolapse patients face. There is an added bonus for those watching their weight; fruits and vegetables are relatively low in calories compared to more dense nutrients such as protein and fat. Good sources of complex carbohydrates are such foods as fruits and fruit juices, leafy vegetables, peas, beans, lentils, potatoes, corn, pasta, and whole-grain breads and cereals. Rice and bran are also included in the complex carbohydrate group. Always choose whole-grain products rather than white-flour products, because of the higher nutrient and fiber content.

Twenty percent of your diet should be composed of protein sources. These include fish, poultry, veal, lamb, pork, cheese, milk, yogurt, eggs, peanut butter, dried peas, and legumes. Once again, to limit the amount of fat in your diet, we recommend drinking skim milk, eating very lean cuts of beef, and substituting fish and poultry for red meat whenever possible. In addition, select low-fat cheeses and yogurt, and remove the skin from poultry.

Finally, about 30 percent of your calorie intake should be from fats. Getting enough fat is rarely a problem. In our society it is much more common to have too many fats than to have too few. We want you not only to limit the amount of fat you take in, but also to be careful to choose the correct types of fats. Remember that a high-fat diet predisposes you to fibrocystic breast disease. It is also associated with a greater incidence of cancer of the colon, breast, pancreas, ovaries, prostate, and rectum. Butter and sour cream that you put on your potato are obvious sources of fat. Less obvious sources are those fats that are contained in protein sources such as hot dogs, cold cuts, fried foods, sauces, gravy, and fatty cuts of meat. We suggest holding down the amount of protein-rich food you eat to about eight ounces a day. In doing this, you will automatically limit the amount of fat you take in. The fat that you do use should be from vegetable sources such as corn oil, salad dressings, nuts, and seeds, rather than animal fats such as butter, cream and whole-milk dairy products, meat fat, and bacon.

If you're in the average weight range or even just ten pounds overweight, rather than counting calories, I would recommend that you just achieve a very nutritious, well-balanced food intake and a begin a moderate aerobic exercise program. Over time the weight will stabilize and take care of itself. Here is a list of guidelines for planning your menus:

- Drink plenty of fluids and beverages that limit caffeine, such as decaffeinated tea, decaffeinated coffee, fruit juices.

- Choose corn oil margarine in tubs or other polyunsaturated fats; for your salads use safflower oil, and corn oil; avoid coconut oil and palm oil.

- Choose lean cuts of beef such as tenderloin, chuck, and rump cuts.

- Remove the skin from poultry.

- Choose fish and chicken over beef whenever possible.

- Limit eggs to three per week.

- Eat vegetables raw, steamed, baked, or broiled rather than sauteed or fried.

- Don't overcook, because this reduces the vitamin content.

- Aim for variety in your diet. A salad, for example, should be varied, not only in color, and texture, but in the food types. Mix different types of greens, such as iceberg and romaine lettuce and spinach. Throw in some red cabbage, yellow squash, tomatoes, cucumbers and radishes. You might also add broccoli, cauliflower, green peppers, and onions.

- You can add a protein source to your diet such as some grated cheese or some sliced turkey. Some people like fruit such as raisins or orange slices in their salad.

- Choose skim milk fortified with vitamins A and D.

- Whatever you do, don't skip breakfast. By breakfast time your body has been without fuel since the night before and needs a good meal. In the "Sample Menus" section later in the chapter are well-balanced breakfasts that require very little preparation time. Once again, they should be a good source of fiber, complex carbohydrates, and some protein, but you should limit your fat intake. Your lunch should be your largest meal of good carbohydrate source and some protein. Studies have shown that people have less trouble maintaining their ideal body weight if they eat the bulk of their calories before 2:00 p.m. Europeans eat this way taking their main meal at lunch time and only a light meal at dinner time. This is the highest-energy diet style. There are some lunches in the "Sample Menus" section. You need not follow them exactly — just use them as a guide, substituting similar foods from among your favorites. (Remember the basic principles of eliminating caffeine and sugar, and carbohydrates and lean protein sources, and limiting fat.)

In planning your diet, follow these general guidelines:

Dietary Recommendations For MVP

| • Increase fluid intake | • Eliminate caffeine |
| • Eliminate sugar | • Limit fat intake |

About Fad Diets

Americans are probably the worst in the world about following every fad diet that is written up in the tabloids at the grocery store check-out counter. If you objectively evaluate these, looking at the calorie intake, the nutritional content, and what is required to maintain the diet, most of them are ridiculous. Let's take, for example, one that uses a lot of grapefruit. If you really add up the calories on that diet, you probably consume 500 to 600 calories a day. Sure, you're going to lose weight on 500 to 600 calories a day, but you're going to pay the price. The same holds true for the high-protein and high-fat diets that dramatically limit complex carbohydrates. Your body will probably lose weight, but most of the weight loss will be fluid, which is devastating to MVP patients, and you will also tend to rebound very quickly after getting back to your normal eating patterns. Fad dieting dramatically diminishes the energy stores of the body. This is bad for everyone, but it is particularly devastating for the patient with MVP. I say emphatically and without reservation, avoid all fad diets. There are menus in this chapter for very safe, sensible weight reduction, but the general rule is, choose a very well-balanced, nutritionally complete eating program, limiting your calories to about 1,200 a day. Whatever you do, don't drop to less than 1,000 calories a day, or you will pay the price in your energy levels.

As previously mentioned when our caloric intake is dramatically dropped, our metabolism slows. Rather than slowing your metabolism to starvation levels, it's by far wiser and in the long run much more effective to stick to a well-balanced, sensible eating program and increase your caloric expenditure by a moderate aerobic exercise program.

Weight Reduction for the MVP Patients

Determine at this moment that you will not go on any diet unless you are determined to make long-term changes in your eating patterns. Avoid the diet merry-go-round or yo-yo effect that's going to result in your body composition being fatter than the day you started. In addition to ruining your body composition over time, yo-yo dieting also makes you pay a price in your energy level. You probably have a weight problem to begin with because your MVP symptoms have diminished your energy levels, and fatigue has resulted in less activity, and thus burning fewer calories, than you need to stay slim.

As with everything dealing with mitral valve prolapse, there is no quick fix, no miracle cure. To lose weight healthfully and successfully, you have to follow some sensible rules. Here are some of the basics for the sensible approach to weight reduction with MVP, integrating dietary considerations into your day-to-day life:

1. Eat a well-balanced diet with a variety of foods. This means eating complex carbohydrates (fruits, vegetables, whole wheat and starches); protein, lean meats, and skim dairy products; fats, and corn oil margarine in limited amounts; and lots of fluids at each meal. Remember that carbohydrates are burned first, giving you an energy surge within three to four hours. Proteins are burned slower, and fats are burned during the remaining time before the next meal. Remember the rule of eating at least half of your caloric intake from complex carbohydrate sources.

2. Establish regular eating patterns. Don't skip breakfast. The old adage stressing the importance of three square meals a day has a lot of truth to it. Regular eating promotes sound nutrition through variety and timing of nutrient availability. It prevents the broad fluctuations in blood sugar that result in drops in your energy level. It prevents the stuffed feeling that you get after overeating because you felt starved from not eating for a long time.

3. Eat about 25 percent of your calories for breakfast. Eat about 50 percent at lunch and the remaining 25 percent in the evening. This gives you most of your calories before 2:00 p.m. and also gives you the highest energy level of any diet, preventing you from overloading the body with calories at night when you are not going to be burning many.

4. Increase calorie expenditure while you decrease calorie intake. Remember that one pound of fat is about 3,500 calories. To lose two pounds, or 7,000 calories, weekly, you would have to burn about 1,000 calories above your food intake per day. To achieve this fat weight loss without a tremendous amount of increased physical activity would probably sap your energy stores. A much more realistic and healthful goal is to lose about one pound per week. You can lose this by decreasing your caloric intake 200 to 300 calories a day below the requirements for daily living and increasing your daily physical activity.

5. Limit the fatty foods in your diet. The ones you should limit include butter, margarine, fried foods, mayonnaise, oils, sauces, salad dressings, avocados, nuts, olives, granola, party crackers, dips, fast foods, convenience foods, pastry, fatty meats (such as bacon, sausage and cold cuts), marbled beef, lamb, pork, and dairy products that are high in fat, such as sour cream, whole milk, most cheeses, and ice cream. Substitute low fat dairy products, low-fat yogurt, and low-fat cheeses. Choose foods like chicken, turkey, or tuna instead of hamburgers and cold cuts. Keep in mind that each gram of fat that you eat contains twice the number of calories as a gram of protein or carbohydrate. Carbohydrate is your bargain food.

6. Eliminate sugar. You will find that sugar sources such as table sugar, honey, jam, jelly, soft drinks, desserts, cookies, candy, pastries, cakes, and sweetened juices stimulate your appetite for more sugar and are essentially nutrient deficient. They are, in other words, empty calories. Learn to read labels. Sugar may be called sucrose, glucose, dextrose,

fructose or lactose, but it's still sugar. Limit to no more than two sweet desserts a week. Substitute fresh fruit instead.

7. Eat high-fiber foods that are low in calories and high in volume. Eat raw fruits and vegetables including the peels and seeds as well, when possible. Baked potatoes, whole-grain cereals, bread, bran, oatmeal, popcorn, broth-based soups, and pasta (if you limit the amount of fatty topping you put on it) are real dieter's bargain. Try fresh pasta with just a spoonful of olive oil and some freshly grated parmesan cheese.

8. Choose lean meats, poultry and fish instead of red meat. It is especially important to weight the meat part of your diet heavily in favor of poultry, fish, and veal. Dramatically limit beef, lamb, and pork. When you do eat beef, concentrate on the leaner cuts such as tenderloin, flank, and round.

9. Prepare foods in a way that dramatically limits the use of fat. Broil or bake meats on a rack, draining off the fat. For gravies use meat drippings with the fat skimmed. Saute foods in water (using a wok, for example), steam vegetables, or eat them raw. Use fat-free butter substitutes such as butter-flavored granules. Try herbs and spices, low-calorie nonstick cooking sprays, and butter-flavored extract. You can buy a basket for cooking on the grill, spray it with a nonstick cooking spray, and use it for grilling fish. Try rubbing a small amount of olive oil on your fish, and then sprinkle blackening seasoning on it; it is absolutely marvelous!

10. Limit alcohol. Remember that MVP patients are extremely sensitive to alcoholic beverages because first, alcohol is a drug, and second these beverages are high in yeast, an allergen to which many people are sensitive. In addition, alcohol calories are empty calories. There are about 150 calories in a two-ounce cocktail, and there is very little nutritive value.

11. Substitute low-calorie snacks such as raw fruit and vegetables, unbuttered popcorn, tomato juice, and salads.

12. Drink six to eight glasses of fluid each day. Remember that water is still the best drink, but you can also drink decaffeinated coffee and tea, low-fat milk, unsweetened fruit juices, low-salt soups, and caffeine-free low-calorie diet drinks.

13. Eat slowly in a pleasant environment. Resolve that you are going to enjoy your food, and plan a time that is just for eating. Don't eat standing in the

kitchen, Set the table, sit down, and chew your food thoroughly. Take at least 20 minutes to finish your meal. It takes about 20 minutes for the brain to get the signals from the increasing blood sugar that it is "time to stop eating." So if you eat slowly, you're less likely to overeat.

14. Choose crunchy foods instead of soft foods. Crunchy foods like apples take longer to chew, and therefore are more satisfying. Also, psychologically we need to chew to relieve stress and tension. Dentists tell us that often prolapse patients under stress grind their teeth. Chewing crunchy foods helps to relieve the stress and eliminate grinding your teeth at night.

15. Preplan your meals. Avoid eating in response to impulse just because you're tired. What you eat on impulse, is usually high-calorie, low-nutrient food. Plan meals carefully, and plan strategies to prevent emotions and moods from interfering with sensible eating. Plan ahead for weekends, holidays, and vacations so they won't interfere with your weight-loss goals.

16. Try to break the snack habit! Remember food is not love. Food is simply fuel for the body. Choose the highest-quality fuel that you can possibly choose.

17. Check with your doctor to see if you need to limit salt intake. As previously mentioned, many MVP patients have low blood pressure and do not need to limit salt. If, however, you do not have low blood pressure sometimes or if you tend to have high blood pressure sometimes, you might need to limit the amount of salt in your diet by limiting pickles, olives, luncheon meats, bacon, sausage, cheeses, and processed foods. Amazingly, many diet drinks are high in salt. Remember that the average American consumes approximately 20 times more salt than is required by the body. So even if you eat some of the foods listed above, try not to salt food at the table.

18. Pay attention to external food cues. Often people who overeat are very sensitive to external cues such as seeing food or smelling food or having extra servings in a bowl on the table. Limit these cues dramatically. Don't combine TV or reading with your eating. Simply eat and enjoy your meal time. If you are distracted while you're eating, you tend to eat more. Keep unneeded food out of the house or certainly out of sight.

19. Perhaps most important is to incorporate more activity into your daily schedule. Certainly a regular exercise program is critical for all of us, and I have outlined this in the chapter on exercise. In addition, remember that calories are burned not only at exercise sessions, but in all sorts of activities that you do throughout the day. Try parking your car a block or two farther away from work. The benefits of walking this extra distance every day will add up. Take the stairs instead of an elevator. Build activities into your daily life that will accumulate over a year. Many of our prolapse patients find that scheduling their exercise session in the late afternoon helps them handle the pressures of the evening meal a lot better. Exercise decreases the appetite and also reaffirms your healthful habits and makes you less likely to overeat at night. But do plan your exercise session for whenever your energy level is high.

20. Try some stress management classes. If you can find a way to manage stress effectively without food or alcohol, problems with overeating and drinking can often be eliminated.

21. Establish life-long eating and exercise habits that will enable you to maintain permanent weight control. This is the heart of the comprehensive approach to weight control that I recommend to my patients. The ultimate goal should be to take off pounds slowly and steadily and make lifestyle changes that enable you to keep them off. A simple but highly effective way of monitoring your progress is to weigh regularly. Don't ever allow yourself to gain more than 2 to 3 pounds above your ideal weight before going back on your weight-reducing formula.

These are some of the most important basic principles for maintaining high energy and ideal body weight. The goal is a lifelong healthful eating plan that will enable you to feel your best and look your best. When you begin to eat sensibly, your energy levels will soar and you'll lay a firm foundation to get involved with enjoyable aerobic activities.

Food Records

Keeping food records may be time consuming and cumbersome at first, but it will help you establish good, solid eating habits. This will dramatically improve your energy levels and enable you to undertake an aerobic conditioning program to help maximize your potential and eliminate the long-standing fatigue so common with MVP.

After a week of keeping your food records, review them objectively. Are you eating adequate amounts of protein? How about complex carbohydrates? Is your fluid intake adequate? What type of fat is common in your diet? Is your caloric intake adequate or excessive? Now that you have that information, try to develop a plan for next week's meals that will be an improvement in all of the important areas. Stick with your plan, and continue to keep records. Check on the record of how you were feeling when you ate. Were you eating for reasons other than hunger? If so, try to think of some strategies to combat stress eating. When good eating becomes a way of life, you will look and feel your best and your body will have the proper fuel to keep you at your peak.

Use the food records on the following pages as you try the menus and recipes that complete this chapter.

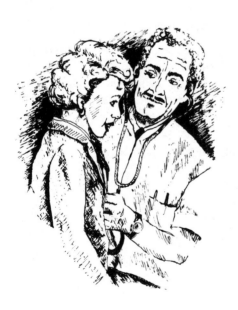

Daily Food Record

	Kind/Amount	How Are You Feeling?
Breakfast		
Lunch		
Dinner		
Snacks		

Date _____

(Make copies of this Record for your daily use.)

SAMPLE MENU NO. 1

For Maintenance for The Average Woman

BREAKFAST
1/2 cup unsweetened fruit juice
1 poached egg
2 slices whole-wheat toast with 1 tsp. corn oil margarine
1 cup skim milk
        Total calories: 375

LUNCH
Tuna salad sandwich
2 slices whole-wheat bread
1/2 cup water-packed tuna with 2 tsp. mayonnaise, lemon juice, pickle,
    and lettuce
1 cup of coleslaw with lemon juice and vinegar
1 medium apple
        Total calories: 435

SUPPER
3 oz. broiled chicken or fish
1 small baked potato with 1 tsp. tub margarine
2 whole-wheat dinner rolls
1/2 cup fresh carrots
1/2 cup spinach
1 cup tossed salad with mixed greens and tomato and 1 tsp. oil and vinegar dressing
1/2 cup fresh or canned unsweetened pineapple chunks
1 cup skim milk
        Total calories for the day: 1,515

SAMPLE MENU NO. 2

For Maintenance for the Average Woman

BREAKFAST
1/2 small banana
3/4 cup dry whole-wheat cereal with 1 cup skim milk
1 slice whole-wheat toast with 1 tsp. tub margarine
          Total calories: 360

LUNCH
1 cup vegetable soup
1/2 cup low-fat cottage cheese
1 cup fresh fruit salad, including citrus fruit
1 whole-wheat muffin with 1 tsp. margarine
1 tomato in wedges
Sliced cucumber with mint, dill, vinegar, and a tsp. of oil
          Total calories: 440

SUPPER
3 oz. baked fish, cooked with 1/2 cup onions and mushrooms, and lemon
1 large ear of corn with 1 tsp. tub margarine
2 whole-wheat dinner rolls
1 cup tossed vegetable salad with lemon-vinegar dressing
1/2 cup zucchini
1 fresh nectarine
          Total calories for the day: 1,510

SAMPLE MENU NO. 1

For Weight Reduction

BREAKFAST
1/2 cup unsweetened orange juice
1 poached egg
1 slice whole-wheat toast with 1 tsp. tub margarine
                Total calories: 225

LUNCH
1 cup vegetable soup
Tuna salad sandwich with 2 slices of whole-wheat bread
        1/2 cup water-packed tuna, and 1 tsp. mayonnaise
1 cup skim milk
1 small apple
                Total calories: 495

SUPPER
2 oz. broiled skinless chicken
1 small baked potato with 1 tsp. tub margarine
1/2 cup fresh carrots
1/2 cup fresh green beans
1 cup tossed lettuce, tomato, and cucumber salad with herb-vinegar
        dressing
                Total calories for the day: 1,005

SAMPLE MENU NO. 2

For Weight Reduction

BREAKFAST
1/2 grapefruit
1/2 cup hot oatmeal with cinnamon and
     1 tsp. tub margarine
1 cup skim milk
          Total calories: 220

LUNCH
Seafood creole with 2 oz. mixed seafood cooked in
     1/2 cup tomato sauce with diced pepper, onion,
     and celery, and served with 1/2 cup rice
1 cup tossed salad with vinegar dressing
          Total calories: 425

SUPPER
2 oz. roast chicken
1/2 cup wild rice
1/2 cup green beans
1/2 cup raisin-carrot salad
1 small baked apple with cinnamon
          Total calories for the day: 1,010

Favorite Personal Recipes

Here are just a few of my favorite recipes. Keep in mind the rules of good nutrition when you create your own favorites. Remember to avoid sugar and substitute low-fat ingredients whenever possible.

Bean Dip

1 can (16 oz.) kidney beans, drained and rinsed
2 tbsp. finely chopped green chiles
1 tbsp. vinegar
1 tsp. chili powder
1/8 tsp. minced onion
2 tsp. parsley

Place all ingredients in a blender and blend until smooth. Serve with fresh vegetables or chips.

Hummus

1 large onion, finely chopped
2 cloves garlic, minced
1 tbsp. corn oil
2 cups cooked garbanzo beans, drained and rinsed
1/2 cup fresh lemon juice
1 tbsp. soy sauce
salt to taste
1/4 cup tahini
1/2 cup sesame seeds, toasted and ground

Cook onion and garlic in the oil until clear. Transfer all ingredients to a blender and process until smooth. Great with chips, or with pita bread for a low-fat sandwich.

Salsa

2 medium tomatoes, chopped
1/2 cup chopped scallions
2 tbsp. chopped hot pepper
1 tbsp. wine vinegar
1 tbsp. vegetable oil

Combine all ingredients and chill for several hours before serving with chips.

Monterey Jack Squares

3 eggs
1/4 cup plus 2 tbsp. all-purpose flour
3/4 tsp. baking powder
1/4 tsp. salt
1-1/2 cup shredded Monterey Jack cheese
1 cup plus 2 tbsp. low-fat cottage cheese
1 can (4 oz.) diced green chiles, drained
Vegetable cooking spray

Beat eggs with mixer 3 minutes. Combine flour, baking powder, and salt; add to eggs and beat until smooth. Stir in cheese and chiles. Pour into 9-inch square baking pan coated with vegetable spray. Bake at 350 degrees for 30--35 minutes. Cool for 10 minutes before serving. Cut into squares.

Spinach-Vegetable Dip

1 cup low-fat sour cream
1/2 cup reduced-calorie mayonnaise
1/2 cup chopped green onion
1 10-oz. package frozen spinach, thawed
1 package leek soup mix
1 tbsp. Italian dressing mix
1 small package slivered almonds

Combine all ingredients and chill for several hours before serving with fresh vegetables or whole-wheat crackers.

Cranberry Punch

4 cups fresh cranberries
1 quart unsweetened apple juice
1 quart water
2 tbsp. grated orange rind
6 cinnamon sticks
12 whole cloves
1 quart unsweetened orange juice

Wash berries and drain. Combine all ingredients except orange juice and simmer 5 minutes. Strain punch and add orange juice. Reheat and serve warm.

Oatmeal Snack Cakes

1-1/4 cups quick-cooking oats, uncooked
1/2 cup chopped dates
1/2 cup raisins
1/4 cup whole-bran cereal
1/2 cup unsweetened crushed pineapple, undrained
1 medium apple, chopped
1 egg
1 tbsp. reduced-calorie margarine
1-1/2 tsp. baking powder
1 tsp. vanilla extract
1/4 tsp. salt
nonstick cooking spray

Combine cereal, raisins, dates, and oats in a large bowl, and set aside. Combine remaining ingredients except cooking spray in electric blender, and blend until smooth. Add this mixture to dry ingredients, stirring until blended. Spoon batter into muffin pans coated with spray. Bake at 350 degrees for 35 minutes. (Snack cakes do not rise during baking.)

Spicy Bulgur

1 cup uncooked bulgur wheat
1 can (10-3/4 oz.) chicken broth
3/4 cup water
1/4 tsp. marjoram
2 tbsp. chopped scallions
1 tbsp. minced fresh parsley

Combine all ingredients except onions in saucepan. Simmer on low heat 20 - 25 minutes. Stir in onions.

Stuffed Baked Apples

4 cooking apples
1/4 cup raisins
3/4 cup unsweetened apple juice
1 tsp. lemon juice
1 tsp. liquid margarine
Ground cinnamon

Core each apple, making a large cavity. Arrange apples in baking pan. Fill cavities with raisins. Combine lemon juice and apple juice and pour over apples. Drizzle small amount of margarine into each cavity. Sprinkle with cinnamon. Bake at 350 degrees for 60 minutes.

Chunky Applesauce

4 large cooking apples
1/2 cup apple juice
1/4 tsp. ground cinnamon
1/8 tsp. ground nutmeg

Peel, core, and chop apples. Combine apples and juice in saucepan. Cook, uncovered over medium heat 10 - 15 minutes. Stir in spices and serve warm or chilled.

Lyn's Baked Fruit

1 large can water-packed sliced peaches
1 large can water-packed sliced pears
1 cup chopped dried apricots
1 can dark pitted cherries
1 cup unsweetened applesauce
1 tsp. cinnamon
2 tbsp. soft margarine

Combine all ingredients and pour into oven-proof baking dish. Bake at 350 degrees for 1 hour. Serve warm as a side dish or dessert. Great for the holidays.

Poached Pears

4 ripe pears, peeled and cored
2 cups cranberry juice
1/4 tsp. cinnamon
1/4 tsp. ground cloves
1 tsp. grated orange rind
1/2 tsp. grated lemon rind

Combine all ingredients in a saucepan. Bring to a boil, reduce heat, and simmer for 15 minutes. Serve the pears warm or chilled. A great dessert following a somewhat heavy meal.

Poached Salmon with Mustard Sauce

1-1/2 cup Chablis
1/2 cup water
1 onion
1 lemon, sliced
4 sprigs parsley
1 tsp. dried dillweed
1/4 tsp. pepper
4 salmon fillets (about 1-1/2 pounds)

Combine all ingredients except fish in skillet. Bring to boil, cover, and simmer for 10 minutes. Add fish fillets and simmer for 8 minutes. Remove fillets to platter and top with mustard sauce.

Mustard Sauce

2 tbsp. margarine
1-1/2 tbsp. flour
1 cup skim milk
1 tsp. dry mustard
1 tsp. lemon juice
1/4 tsp. salt

Melt margarine over low heat; add flour, stirring until smooth. Cook 1 minute. Add milk and cook until thickened. Remove from heat and stir in mustard and lemon juice. Yields 1 cup.

Barbecued Shrimp

2-1/2 pounds large fresh shrimp, peeled
1/2 cup lemon juice
1/4 cup Italian dressing
1/4 cup soy sauce
3 tbsp. minced parsley
3 tbsp. minced onion
1 clove garlic, crushed
1/2 tsp. ground pepper (optional)

Place shrimp in shallow baking dish. Combine remaining ingredients in a jar, cover, and shake vigorously. Pour over shrimp. Cover and refrigerate for at least 4 hours. Thread shrimp onto skewers. Broil or grill 5 to 6 inches from medium heat 3 to 4 minutes on each side, basting frequently. Serves 6.

Lyn's Greek Snapper

2 large snapper fillets
1/4 cup soft margarine
1/4 cup lemon juice
1 lemon, sliced
4 cloves garlic, crushed
1 tsp. oregano
1/4 tsp. paprika

Place snapper in shallow aluminum pan (disposable is great). In a saucepan combine remaining ingredients and simmer for 3 minutes. Pour over snapper and refrigerate for 4 hours. Place pan on outdoor barbecue grill (medium heat for gas grill or small charcoal fire). Cook for 10 to 12 minutes, basting frequently. Do not turn. Serves 2 to 4 depending on the size of the fillets.

Cheesy Wine Chicken

4 chicken breasts with bones
1 can cheddar cheese soup
1 can (use the empty soup can) white wine
Combine the wine and soup, pour over chicken, and bake at 350 degrees for 1 hour.

Parmesan Oven Fried Chicken

1/2 cup fine bread crumbs
1/3 cup grated parmesan cheese
1 tbsp. chopped parsley
1/4 tsp. garlic salt
1/4 tsp. pepper
6 chicken breast halves, skinned
1/4 cup Italian dressing

Combine first five ingredients; set aside. Dip chicken in salad dressing; dredge in bread-crumb mixture. Place chicken in baking pan coated with cooking spray. Bake at 350 degrees for 45 minutes or until tender.
Serves 6.

Orange Spinach Salad

3/4 pound fresh spinach leaves, torn
1 can mandrin orange slices
1 small package sliced almonds, toasted
1/4 cup reduced-calorie Italian dressing

Combine first three ingredients in salad bowl. Pour dressing over salad and toss.

Tabouleh

1 cup bulgur wheat
2 cups boiling water
1 large tomato, chopped
1/2 cup minced fresh parsley
1/4 cup chopped green onion
1 tbsp. minced fresh mint
1/4 cup lemon juice
1 tbsp. olive oil
1/4 tsp. salt
1/4 tsp. pepper

Combine bulgur and water; let stand 1 hour. Drain, add remaining ingredients, and mix well. Refrigerate overnight. Spoon onto lettuce leaves to serve. Makes 8 servings.

Potato Soup

4 medium potatoes, peeled and cubed
1 large onion, chopped
3 cups water
1 cup milk
1 tsp. salt
1 tsp. chicken-flavored bouillon
2 tsp. chives
1/8 tsp. pepper
1/4 cup sliced carrots
1/4 cup broccoli flowers

Combine potatoes, onion, and water in saucepan. Bring to boil; cover and simmer for 15 minutes. Add carrots and broccoli; simmer 8 more minutes. Add milk and spices. Serves 6.

Artichokes Supreme

2 cans artichoke hearts, chopped
1 cup reduced-calorie mayonnaise
1 cup parmesan cheese
1 tsp. garlic salt

Gently combine ingredients and bake for 20 minutes in 375 degree oven, or heat in microwave on medium power for 3 to 5 minutes. Can be used as a vegetable side dish or as a great dip for crackers.

6 The Role of Medication in the Management of MVP

I debated as to whether or not I should even include a chapter on medication in this text. I believe that I must do so for completeness, but I also realize that it may lead to problems, because some individuals may be looking for a recipe they can take to a physician and say "See here, she recommends Brand X, and you haven't prescribed that." Please, please realize that I do not prescribe or even recommend medications. That can only be done by a physician. I can only share with you information regarding some of the medications that I see frequently used for MVP, their indications, and their side effects.

May I say again, and emphatically, it is better if MVP symptoms can be controlled without medication not to take anything whatsoever. Medication should be used only as directed by your physician and should not be adjusted by you according to your daily symptoms. Never take medication that has been prescribed for someone else. A physician evaluates each individual's situation and chooses a medication appropriately. Even if your neighbor has symptoms similar to yours, there may be some specific reasons why your physician would recommend a different medication.

Looking For Short Cuts

One major difficulty in our culture today is the tendency to look for short cuts. We want magic, instantaneous cures that require no effort on our part. We are, unfortunately, a drug-oriented culture. This is not limited to youth. Many adults reach for a legal drug, alcohol, on a daily basis for the relaxation that it can provide. Others use alcohol when they are in tense social situations to bolster their confidence. Still others reach for medication to sleep every night. Caffeine is another socially acceptable drug that is widely used and abused in our adult society. Many of these same adults would be incensed if you accused them of drug abuse. The idea I am trying to get across is that in our culture we have begun to look for the quick fix, the easy way out, and to assume that if we seek out a physician, he or she can give us some special potion that will solve all of our problems. This is not true, least of all for MVP. Good diet, exercise, positive mental attitude, and in general a healthy approach to taking control of one's life are what we need. If all these measures are not enough, certainly we need to seek some medication. But medication alone is not enough to control this syndrome. I have had numerous patients return on their six-week follow-up visit saying that they were feeling some better but not quite well. When questioned, they indicated that they were not exercising or following the proper dietary guidelines but they were taking their medication exactly as prescribed. It simply is not enough.

Medication Resistant Individuals

Some individuals are very resistant to taking any type of medication whatsoever. A typical example is the individual who comes to me after several years of symptoms and who has had multiple unsuccessful interactions with numerous physicians. Her illness has progressed to the point that she has virtually every symptom in the book as well as severe social avoidance (agoraphobia) and almost constant panic attacks. She comes in and says "I am desperate for help, but I don't want to take any medication. I have tried several things, but they don't work, and I don't want to try anything else." While I can appreciate the notion of having a healthy respect for all medicines and not wanting to take medication excessively, I also realize that there are many conditions that require the prudent use of medications carefully chosen for the particular situation. Patients must have enough trust in the professionals they have sought to give their recommendations a fair trial. It often requires several weeks of taking medication to begin to notice improvements. Be patient, and continue to follow the lifestyle recommendations in the previous chapters.

Self Medication

A third frequently encountered problem associated with medication is the self-medicator, an individual who adjusts the dosage in response to changes in symptoms from day to day. Such patients increase dosage if they happen to be feeling poorly and decrease dosage on good days. They also tend to take medication either prescribed for someone else with similar problems or prescribed for themselves at a different time, perhaps by a different doctor. Beware! Just as an attorney who represents himself has a fool for a client, a patient who medicates himself has a fool for a patient. There are a number of drug interactions that can be quite harmful. The whole idea in the treatment of MVP is balance--balance of the autonomic nervous system. In order to be effective, medication has to be taken as prescribed and continued until balance is achieved. Harm can also come from abruptly discontinuing medications. Do not suddenly stop taking medication simply because your symptoms have improved. Check with your doctor first! Medication for MVP is rarely needed for extended periods of time (years), but it is not uncommon to require medication for several months.

Sometimes, although a medication is carefully chosen and you still may experience uncomfortable side effects. You need to communicate with your doctor so that he or she can adjust the dosage or change the medication. The doctor may tell you that with a particular medication certain side effects are expected at first but that they usually resolve in a few days and that the benefits you can experience should outweigh the initial discomfort. If this happens, give the medication a fair try before you insist on discontinuing it.

Never mix medications prescribed by more than one doctor. If Dr. A prescribes a drug and Dr. B prescribes another, be sure to check with Dr. B about whether he wants you to continue with your initial medication or to switch to the new medication alone. Along the same lines, MVP patients tend to have several specialists working on their case at the same time. All specialists may be quite competent and doing a great job with their parts of your care. But you still need a primary physician, a doctor who is coordinating the efforts of this group, so that you will not have treatment plans that are in conflict with one another. Your internist, family physician, gynecologist, or cardiologist could serve as primary physician. Be sure to keep him or her informed of other physicians' recommendations.

Medications Frequently Used For MVP

The medications listed on the following page in Table 6-1 are frequently used in the treatment of MVP.

Table 6-1. Medications Frequently Used for MVP

Beta Blocking Agents

Blocadran	Lopressor
Corgard	Tenoretic
Corzide	Tenormin
Inderal	Timolide
Inderide	Visken
Kerlone	

Calcium Channel Blockers

Calan	Isoptin
Cardizem	Procardia

Antimigraine Agents

Cafegot	Sansert
Ergostat	Wigraine
Midrin	

Antidepressants

Adapin	Ludiomil
Amitriptyline	Nardin
Asendin	Norpramine
Aventyl	Pamelor
Deprol	Parnate
Desyrel	Prozac
Elavil	Sinequan
Endep	Tofranil
Etrafon	Triavil
Librium	Vivactil
Limbitrol	

Antianxiety Agents

Ativan	Tranzene
Librium	Valium
Serax	Xanax
Klonopin	

Miscellaneous Medications

Clonodine

The list is by no means exhaustive. New drugs are being released every day. Instead of discussing each drug in detail I will try to familiarize you with the basic classifications of drugs. I have also included in this section a listing of medications that can be purchased over the counter without a prescription that contain caffeine, ephedrine, pseudoephedrine, phenylephrine, and phenoylpropanolamine, substances that can aggravate the symptoms of MVP by increasing heart rate. Because heart rate changes are uncomfortable for MVP patients, these medications could be problematic. If in doubt about buying a medication over the counter without a prescription, ask your pharmacist.

Beta Blockers

Beta blockers are a specific class of drugs. Often used to slow heart rate and to control blood pressure. Their name reflects the fact they act on certain types of cells, known as beta cells, that are common in the heart and in the blood vessels. Examples of beta blockers are Inderal (propranolol hydrochloride), Tenormin (atenolol), and many others. Table 6-1 lists many of the common beta blockers. Beta blockers are often thought of as "cardiac" or "heart" drugs, but they actually have many uses. A few common uses in the MVP population include control of rapid heartbeat, chest pain, blood pressure, and vascular (migraine) headaches. Each different beta blocker acts a little bit differently. If you have had a bad experience with one of these drugs, you may be able to tolerate others very well.

All beta blockers have some side effects, but some have fewer than others. Your physician may need to try several to find one that is effective for you without excessive side effects. The most commonly mentioned side effects include excessively slow heart rate, fatigue, depression, insomnia, gastrointestinal distress, and exacerbation of asthma symptoms. Low blood pressure may also occur. Beta blockers are often used in patients with MVP who experience rapid heartbeat or those with many extra or skipped beats. They are, however, not appropriate for all patients. and care should be taken to evaluate the patient's particular situation prior to choosing a beta blocker. **Patients with asthma or numerous allergies often do not tolerate beta blockers. Check with your physician.**

Calcium Channel Blockers

The exact mechanisms of action of calcium channel blockers are still being defined. They are believed to dilate coronary arteries as well as some arteries in the extremities, thereby reducing spasm of these arteries. They also produce an increase in exercise tolerance, probably by reducing the heart's demand for oxygen (this is done by decreasing the heart rate and blood pressure). In Table 6-1 I list a number of commonly used calcium channel blockers. They may be used to control chest pain and may also be tried to help improve the fatigue that is common with MVP. Side effects include excessively low blood pressure and heart rate. Other rare side effects include flushing, dizziness, and insomnia.

Medications For Migraine Headaches

Anyone who experiences migraine headaches knows how miserable they can be. Migraine headaches are characterized by severe pain usually on one side of the head. Often there is a sensation known as an *aura* that is noticed just prior to the onset of the headache. Migraines may be accompanied by nausea and an extreme sensitivity to light. The source of these headaches is thought to be the abnormal contraction and dilation of the blood vessels in the brain. Migraine headaches are seen in both sexes, but more often in females. Migraines are most common in individuals 20 to 45 years old. Table 6-1 lists a number of headache medications. Care must be taken with the MVP patient to avoid preparations such as Cafergot that contain caffeine. In small doses, antidepressants may be very effective in controlling migraine headaches. This is because of their effect on the central nervous system.

Other Medications Used For MVP

Table 6-2 list caffeine-containing, over-the-counter medications. The list may be helpful when you are looking for medications for colds and hay fever for example.

Often patients with MVP find that they must take other types of medications, such as blood pressure medications or allergy medications. Space does not allow a full discussion of every situation or every medication. Instead, make sure that the physician prescribing the medication is familiar with your medical history and is aware of your MVP and whatever medication you are taking. Certain types of dysautonomia may respond to medications that may seem somewhat unusual. For example, if the parasympathetic nervous system is too active, the person may experience irritable bowel syndrome as well as other more typical prolapse symptoms such as bradycardia (slow heartbeat) and panic attacks. Medications such as Donnatal may be used to treat this type of dysautonomia.

Antibiotics may be recommended for patients with MVP undergoing dental work and for other types of procedures that might introduce bacteria into the blood stream. The prolapsed valve is at a slightly higher risk of infection than the

Table 6-2. Over-the-Counter Medications the MVP Patient Should Avoid

Caffeine-Containing Over-the-Counter Drugs
    Anacin (Whitehall Labs)
    Anacin Maximum Strength
    Anorexin Capsules (Thompson)
    Appedrine Tablets (Thompson)
    Aqua-Ban (Thompson Medical)
    Ayd's Extra Strength (Jeffrey Martin)
    Ayd's am/pm (Jeffrey Martin)
    Caffedrine Capsule (Thompson Medical)
    Caltrim Reducing Plan Tablets (Commerce)
    DeWitt Pills (DeWitt)
    Dexatrim Capsules (Thompson)
    Doan's Pills (Jeffrey Martin)
    Excedrin Extra-Strength Tablets and Capsules (Bristol-Myers)
    Extra-Strength Dexatrim
    Goody's Extra-Strength Tablets and Powders
    Gold Medal Diet Caps (Pfeiffer)
    Midol Maximum Strength (Glenbrook)
    Midol
    PAC (Upjohn)
    Prolamine Capsules
    Panodyne's Analgesic (Keystone)
    Odrinex Tablets (Fox)
    Quick-Pep Tablets (Thompson Medical)
    Spantrol Capsules (North American)
    Thinz Span, Thinz Back to Nature
    Trigesic
    Wakoz (Jeffrey Martin)
    Vanquish Caplet
    Summit
    Vivarin Tablets (Beecham)
    Wakoz (Jeffrey Martin)

Epinephrine-Containing Over-the-Counter Drugs

Asthma Haler	Bronitin Mist
Asthma Nefrin	Bronkaid Mist
Breath Easy	Medihaler-Epi
Vaponefrin	Insect sting kits
Primatene Mist solution and suspension	

Table 6-2. Over-the-Counter Medications the
MVP Patient Should Avoid (Continued)

Ephedrine-Containing Over-the-Counter Drugs
Histadyl EC   Quelidrin
Quiet Nite   NyQuil

Pseudoephedrine-Containing Over-the-Counter Drugs
Actifed Tabs, Caps, and Liquid
Ambenyl-D
Chlor-trimeton Decongestant
CoTylenol Decongestant Liquid, Tabs, and Caps
Cosanyl
Cosanyl DM
Fedahist Expectorant and Syrup
Fedrazil
Dimacol Liquid and Capsules
Dorcol
Noratuss II
Novafed, Novafed A
Novahistine Cough and Cold Formula
Novahistine DMX
Novahistine Expectorant
Pediacare 2 Liquid
Pediacare 3 Liquid
Pediacare 3 Chewable Tablets
Robatussin DAC
Robatussin PE
Ryna-C
Ryna-CX
Ryna Liquid
Sudafed, Sudafed Plus
Sudafed Cough Syrup
Viromet Tablets

Prescription Drugs Containing Caffeine
Cafergot (for migraine headache)
Fiorinal (for headache)
Soma Compound (pain relief)
Darvon Compound (pain relief)

normally shaped valve. Infection is quite rare, but when it does occur, it can be quite serious. For this reason many physicians recommend antibiotics for dental and other procedures. Many other physicians do not recommend antibiotics, believing that the risk of infection is so low that it does not justify the risk of a reaction that can occur in some individuals taking antibiotics. Table 6-3 shows recent recommendations for antibiotic prophylaxis. These recommendations change frequently. You should check with your physician regarding his/her recommendations.

Recommended Antibiotic Regimens For Procedures

Oral regimen for patients not allergic to Penicillin: Penicillin V — 2.0 Grams orally one hour before, and then 1.0 grams six hours after procedure.

Oral regimen for penicillin-allergic patients: Erythromycin — 1.0 grams, orally one hour before, and then 500 milligrams six hours after procedure.

Table 6-3. Antibiotic Prophylaxis

Procedures That May Require Antibiotic Prophylaxis

All dental procedures likely to induce gum bleeding (not simple adjustment of orthodontic appliances or loss of deciduous teeth)

Tonsillectomy or adenoidectomy

Surgical procedures or biopsy involving the respiratory system

Bronchoscopy

Incision and drainage of infected tissue (abscess, etc.)

Procedures involving the urinary tract (cystoscopy, etc)

Procedures involving the esophagus, stomach, or bowel (endoscopy)

Vaginal gynecological procedures

Gallbladder surgery

Irritable Bowel Syndrome

Donnatal is one of a number of medications that may be used for irritable bowel syndrome. Your best bet is to check with your physician for the control of irritable bowel symptoms.

General Recommendations

Once again, take the medication prescribed by your doctor. Never take medication that was prescribed for someone else. Take the exact dosage the doctor recommends; do not change the dosage on a daily basis to cope with symptoms unless your physician has specifically instructed you to do so. Do not discontinue medication without first checking with your physician.

7 The Role of Positive Mental Attitude in the Management of MVP

There is no way that I can overemphasize the importance of positive mental attitude in patients dealing with the symptoms of MVP. The mind is extremely powerful, probably more powerful than any of us realize. I will not attempt in one chapter to reproduce the wealth of literature on the necessity of positive mental attitude. I have, however, provided many sources of this information in the "Suggested Reading" section at the end of the book.

Stress plays a very important role in the development of peptic ulcer disease, heart disease, high blood pressure, ulcerative colitis, and many other health problems that we see in almost epidemic proportions in modern society. As previously mentioned, it is not at all uncommon to find that a stressful event has triggered the onset of symptoms of MVP. Once again, the stressor need not be emotional in origin, such as the death of a loved one or a divorce; it can also be a physical stressor, such as an operation, childbirth, an automobile accident, or a bad viral illness. The body does not seem to be able to differentiate between stress from an emotional source and stress from a physical source. It perceives any stress as an insult to the body, regardless of its cause.

One particularly interesting study of the biochemical results of stress was conducted on workers in a large aircraft factory in Germany. People in this factory were subjected to noise stress. Every day, for large portions of the work day, there was very loud noise. Noise stress is easy to measure (or quantify) and study. Researches made a number of chemical measurements on these employees before they began work at the aircraft factory and a few months later, after they had been subjected to the noise stress. They found that certain biochemical events happened after prolonged stress, and that many of the employees were beginning to experience fatigue, shortness of breath, diminished exercise capacity, and anxiety. These are not unlike MVP symptoms. For this reason, we have done some similar measurements of some of the biological parameters in MVP patients and found that, indeed, some of the very same biochemical markers were there. The symptoms you experience are biochemical in their origin.

Don't Be A "Yesbut"

A "yesbut" personality is very common among MVP patients. I can quickly identify yesbuts as I am discussing suggestions with them for altering their lifestyle or perhaps taking medication. Their answer is "Yes but I know this won't work for me." These people have become locked into negative thinking because of weeks, months, or even years of poor experiences with the health care delivered for their condition. It is understandable that this should happen. They have tried a number of things that have failed. However, I would encourage you to put failures behind you. Be open to new suggestions, or even the same suggestions combined in a little bit different way. Positive mental attitude is absolutely essential to overcoming some of the problems you are currently experiencing. I can understand that if a person has been to a dozen physicians, tried dozens of kinds of medication, and is still getting progressively worse, he or she can come in with a certain cynical outlook on everything. However, you are doomed to fail if you walk in with that attitude. After evaluating a person's prior experience with health care, we try to make an initial evaluation before any diagnostic testing is performed and to evaluate whether the person is emotionally ready to wipe the slate clean and start fresh with a new approach to the problem. We encourage people to accept the program with enthusiasm and a hopeful attitude. We have group sessions every week to encourage this approach.

Books can help, too. These "rah-rah" books that fill my bookshelves deal with "pulling one's own strings," "being one's own best friend," and "the importance of positive mental attitude." Although I do not have MVP in my own life I have found the approach suggested by these books to be invaluable in overcoming some of the obstacles that we all must face in this hectic world. I would first suggest that you read several of the sources listed in "Suggested Reading" and try to adapt them to your daily living.

Biofeedback

A number of methods may be used to deal with a patient's emotional response to a chronic problem, among them biofeedback. Biofeedback techniques employ some very simple equipment that enables a patient to practice relaxation techniques and see the results. For example, a tiny temperature sensor is clipped onto one of the fingers, and the person is instructed in relaxation technique. As the person relaxes, the blood vessels in the fingers dilate, and thus the temperature at the sensor goes up. This may sound very simple, and it is, but relaxation takes a lot of practice.

I was first involved in biofeedback a number of years ago when I was conducting cardiac rehabilitation classes for patients following open heart surgery or heart attack. These patients found this technique very helpful in learning to relax in their daily lives. As I have previously mentioned, a number of prolapse patients were also referred to me at this same time, and I used this same technique on those patients. Amazingly, those patients found the technique even more helpful than did the heart attack patients, I think, once again, because the patient with MVP has an extremely sensitive nervous system.

We can't eliminate all stress in our lives. It is part of our society, part of our world. We can, however, change the way we respond to stress and the way we allow it to affect our bodily functions and processes. Biofeedback can be used to help diffuse stress in the work place or in the home, and it can also be used as an excellent tool for relaxation and sleep problems.

Other Relaxation Techniques

Relaxation techniques can be very helpful to almost everyone in every lifestyle. In learning to teach these techniques in our cardiac rehabilitation program, I have also come to use them daily in my own personal life to relax in between appointments, to sleep after a particularly stressful day, or to energize myself before a situation I expect to be extremely stressful.

There are a number of good sources of information about relaxation techniques in "Suggested Reading." Many of them use the technique of imagery. Imagery consists of relaxing by imagining a particularly pleasant, relaxing scene. The scene varies for every individual. One person imagines herself at the seashore, lying on the warm sand, listening to the sound of the waves, watching sailboats on the horizon. Another person may imagine himself in the mountains, in a cabin watching the snow fall, sitting in front of a fire. Whatever is particularly helpful for you should be your scene. We are all capable of using our imaginations. Unfortunately our culture has come to rely on stimulation from external sources, such as television sets and radios. But we can still receive a great deal of pleasure from simply using our minds to imagine pleasant, relaxing things and allowing our bodies to respond to these relaxing images and diffuse the stress that is all around us.

Summing Up

In summary, it is critical that the person with prolapse not become a yesbut personality. Make notes for yourself. How often do *you* say, "Yes, but" How often, when you are listening to another individual, are you closed to what he or she is saying, as opposed to being open-minded? Although you may have experienced unpleasant or unsuccessful attempts to control MVP symptoms, you must open yourself to new approaches and allow your powerful mind to assist with the stabilization of your condition.

8 When Panic or Anxiety Attacks — The MVP Connection

Does this scene sound familiar? You're finished with your marketing, and you're heading for the checkout counter. As you approach, you begin to notice that your heart is beating rapidly, you are short of breath, and you have the feeling that you need to run. You attempt to relax, take a deep breath, and shake the feeling, but it will not go away. You're scared. The longer you stand there, the more frightened you become. You can feel your heart beating up into your throat. Your knees are becoming weak, your mouth is dry, your arms are tingling. You think "Am I going to die? Am I going to have a heart attack? I am going to faint and embarrass myself in front of all these people!" You have an almost overwhelming desire to run out of the place. Try as you may, you cannot control these sensations, and suddenly you run from the store, leaving behind all of your groceries and a crowd of people looking at you. You dash home, some how managing to make it there, and you are still frightened and now short of breath. You collapse, terrified and embarrassed. Your pounding heart slowly begins to calm down.

How about this scene? You are sound asleep, and at 2:00 in the morning you are suddenly awakened by a pounding in your chest and a sensation that you are going to smother. You sit bolt upright and become increasingly short of breath. You break out in a cold sweat. You get up from bed pacing back and forth, awakening your husband, telling him that you are frightened. At this point, if it is your first time, he may load you into the car and take you to the emergency room where an EKG is performed, and someone may listen to your chest and then shake his head and say that there's nothing wrong, that it's mitral valve prolapse. No problem. Go home and "learn to live with it," or "get hold of yourself."

These may sound like unusual incidents, but I hear about them all the time. In reality, millions of Americans, predominantly young females, though it can also happen to males, and to people of any age group, suffer from symptoms such as these. Most of my patients do not like to admit to "panic attacks." However, we have found that upon careful questioning many prolapse patients report "spells," "attacks," "smothering sensations," and other symptoms that cause them a great deal of anxiety and make them feel like they are losing control of their bodies or minds. Fully 60 percent of my patients report panic attacks of one variety or another. Panic attacks, for lack of a better term, are accompanied by overwhelming sensations of fear and distress without apparent cause and they are uniformly uncomfortable and upsetting to patients. To the outsider, a panic attack may seem like an unreasonable or neurotic outburst, but the underlying cause for panic disorder is most definitely biological in origin. It may also be genetic, or inherited. In this respect, panic attack or anxiety attack is a disease, just the same as diabetes or arthritis is a disease. But unlike diabetes or arthritis, this disease has a complication called a *phobia* that is a debilitating psychological phenomenon. Phobia means an avoidance, self-imposed limitation on the activities of daily living. For example, the woman who had her first attack in the supermarket, from that day forward, I can assure you, did everything in her power to avoid supermarkets. It is quite clear that panic attacks are not caused by supermarkets, although it is very difficult to convince this lady of that fact. The patient who experiences an anxiety attack on awakening in the middle of the night may thereafter have problems of sleeping. Phobias are the result of a fearful experience. It is a perfectly natural phenomenon when something scares you terribly to avoid anything that you think is going to cause those uncomfortable feelings again.

Dysautonomia and Panic

When people who have dysautonomia, with an already very sensitive nervous system, experience an unpleasant event, such as an episode of rapid heartbeat or an episode of chest pain, their sensitive nervous system perceives this to an exaggerated degree. As a result, their nervous system responds to an exaggerated degree, pouring out adrenalin, which further increases the heart rate, makes the hands cold and clammy, makes breathing come much faster, and gives that sickening "surge of blood" feeling to the head that many of us have experienced. The fear then accelerates, and the patient enters a vicious cycle of fear, physical symptoms, more fear, and uncontrolled terror.

We treat panic and anxiety disorders in a number of ways. Certain types of medications may tend to block the biochemical causes of panic. However, many authorities believe, and I agree, that merely giving medication is not adequate. One must also try to stabilize the autonomic nervous system to prevent the initial triggers such as the rapid heartbeat, the shortness of breath, or the smothering sensation from happening. I also recommend group sessions that teach patients how to control the body's response to an unpleasant trigger. These sessions are invaluable in giving the patient confidence to meet these unpleasant sensations head on and control them.

Panic disorder is classified as a very extreme form of anxiety. *Anxiety* is an uneasy feeling of increased vigilance. (Remember in Chapter 1, the hypervigilance of dysautonomia?) Not all anxiety is bad. It can be good if it prevents us from missing deadlines or falling asleep at the wheel of the car, or helps us escape from the tiger (in our ancestor's day). In fact, a certain amount of anxiety is crucial for our survival as human beings. *Panic*, however, is extremely heightened anxiety. Here is a list of typical symptoms of panic disorder:

Panic Disorder Symptoms

- Shortness of Breath
- Palpitations
- Dizziness
- Smothering
- Unreality Feelings

- Chest Pain
- Faintness
- Sweating
- Fear of Dying
- Intense Impulse to Flee or Seek Help

The physiological (bodily) components of panic — a sudden burst of adrenalin, resulting in increased heart rate, respirations, and blood flow — are closely associated with the "fight or flight" response that enables us to escape the saber-toothed tiger or battle our way through dangerous situations. Arousal or fear, therefore, is a normal and necessary response. Panic can, however, be a serious problem when it comes without any threat from the external environment. People with panic attacks may experience several such attacks in a day, with each episode lasting from 15 minutes to more than an hour. Often patients report palpitations (fluttering heartbeats), dizziness, light-headedness, nausea, smothering, chest pain, choking or an eerie feeling that one is going to die. Even when it is very obvious that there is no external danger to the person, panic and the feelings in the body are extremely frightening to the patient. You could say that a panic attack is much like a faulty smoke alarm that keeps on going off even when there is no smoke or fire in the area. The problem really isn't the noisy alarm itself (the symptoms), but an underlying defect in the trigger or mechanical setting.

Researchers believe that people with panic attacks have an abnormal failure of the biochemical panic trigger in the brain that leaves them vulnerable to recurrent attacks. One line of research centers on a part of the brain that seems to control emotional responses called the *limbic system*. This is closely associated with the autonomic nervous system. The cells in this area are rich in norepinephrine — a brain chemical that helps regulate physiological arousal. Researchers believe that people with panic attacks have some basic metabolic defect that results in an excess production or an oversensitivity to certain chemical messengers in the blood. These messengers enter the specialized part of the brain and in turn trigger the emotional or physical changes of panic.

It is not known at what biochemical point the metabolic failure lies or what sets off the chemical reaction within the brain. But there are some interesting clues. Fatigue following physical illness, alcohol abuse, or drug use, especially cocaine or marijuana, can all exacerbate panic symptoms. All of these chemicals alter brain function. Even common caffeine, used experimentally, can trigger panic attacks in some patients. This is one of the reasons I advise a dramatically limited caffeine intake in prolapse patients. Another chemical that can trigger panic attacks is sodium lactate. Remember that patients with prolapse often have abnormally high lactic acid build-up with exercise. This build-up can actually be a trigger for panic attacks. Panic attack is also worse in females just prior to the menstrual cycle. It is believed that the female hormone progesterone, released during the latter phases of the menstrual cycle, stimulates the same nervous system sites that are so sensitive to caffeine and lactates. We believe this is also why panic attacks are twice as common in women as in men, although, we do often see men with panic attacks. Women with panic disorder tend to have more panic attacks associated with the premenstrual phase than at other times in the menstrual cycle. As I previously mentioned, when men experience panic attacks they tend to experience not only the terror females experience but also an added burden of shame. Remember that panic attacks can make an individual feel out of control, and males tend to feel somewhat emasculated by this condition.

Biochemistry definitely plays a role in the origin of panic attacks, but so do psychological stresses. A recent study by the National Institute of Mental Health, shows that more than 80 percent of people who suffer with panic attacks have experienced an unusually stressful life event not long before their attack. Does this sound familiar? Of my patients with MVP syndrome, 95 percent report a stressful event just prior to the onset of symptoms. As I have mentioned before, the event may involve work, home, or some other source of stress such as a bad viral illness. Men with panic attacks most often report stressful job situations; women with panic attacks most often report interpersonal stressors. Panic attacks occur most frequently in the early 20's, which is often a time of major adjustment from single life to married life or from student to full-time adult responsibilities.

Medications

It is important, if you have panic disorder to understand that outside events are usually not the triggers; that the origins of panic attacks are biochemical and internal. Thus, a self-imposed house arrest with a patient almost unable to leave the safety of the home will just result in an altered lifestyle and rarely control the panic attacks themselves. Panic attacks are now becoming an area of research in psychiatry, psychology, and neurobiology that is quite exciting and offers the hope of some dramatic relief in the near future. Let me say that in almost every case, panic attack can be blocked effectively by the right choice of medication. Furthermore, once the attacks are controlled, the accompanying fear and phobias can be successfully overcome, although it frequently means seeking the help of a psychologist to confront and control these fears.

A number of medications are useful in treating panic disorders. Several of them are listed here, but remember that many medications have adverse effects on the autonomic nervous system. Just because these medications are mentioned, does not necessarily mean that they are recommended for patients with prolapse. The list merely summarizes the results of the most modern research on panic disorder. These medications include:

1. Benzodiazapines. These include Xanax (alprazolam) and Klonopin (clonazepam). These medications can be very effective in blocking panic. They are chemically similar to popular tranquilizers such as Valium (diazepam) and Librium (chlordiazepoxide hydrochloride), which also reduce anxiety but do not stop panic attacks. Benzodiazapines are simple to take and have few side effects, but they can be habit forming.

2. Tricyclic antidepressants. Tofranil (imipramine hydrochloride) was the first drug found to be effective against panic. Its success suggests a possible link between panic disorder and depression. A similar drug is Norpramin, which may also be used to treat panic.

3. Monoamine oxidase (MAO) inhibitors. These drugs include Nardil (phenelzine sulfate) and Parnate (tranylcypromine sulfate). They may provide some relief to people who are resistant to other drugs or cannot, for some reason, take other drugs. It is very important that people who are taking this type of drug avoid certain foods that contain amino acid tyramine, such as aged cheddar cheese, red wine, and pickled and fermented products. These products may interfere with the effectiveness of the drugs, and the combination of drug and amino acid could potentially be harmful.

With all these drugs the aim is to find the minimum effective dosage, because all have certain side effects. Selecting the right drug and the right dosage is not easy. It is a balancing act requiring a physician trained in the use of these medications. If you are put on these medications, you should take them regularly for six to twelve months, after which time the dosage is generally tapered off. But even with effective treatment, panic attack treated with these drugs is not cured, only blocked. This is why one should aim at controlling the triggers to the panic attacks and controlling the person's response to the panic attack. Professional counseling or stress management can help to diffuse the psychological triggers that can lead to subsequent attacks.

Phobias

When panic attacks are diagnosed very early in the course of a person's problem, a trial of drug therapy may be all that is needed to control the symptoms. Unfortunately, most people who experience panic or anxiety attacks do not seek treatment until they have been experiencing the attacks for quite some time. I believe this is because such behavior is labelled as "neurotic." The longer the attacks are allowed to persist, the more likely it is that other symptoms, such as phobias, will develop. Remember the vicious cycle — a frightening trigger, the bodily response, further fear, and the tendency to avoid whatever the person associates with the trigger, such as supermarkets, parties, or sleeping. The emotions that accompany these attacks are often hard to put into words. Many people feel ashamed and say that they are afraid they have "lost control." They begin hiding the very information that would help the doctor pinpoint their problems. When they do seek medical care, it is usually for physical symptoms, which in many cases disappear when the attacks are controlled. People who have suffered panic attacks for a long time tend to have been seen by many doctors in search of relief.

Agoraphobia, fear of open spaces, is a term that is often used to describe the phobic state that grows out of recurrent panic attacks. The person usually develops an overwhelming fear of places or situations that he or she believes might produce a panic attack. This anticipatory fear of places or things can become expanded as more panic attacks occur to include more and more locations. The typical sites for attacks include supermarkets, shopping centers, restaurants, automobiles, parties, bridges, elevators, tunnels, freeways, and airplanes, spaces where there is a perceived threat and where there is very little ability to escape.

Eventually, if not treated, a person with panic disorder can become incapacitated and virtually home bound, because of the fear of having a panic attack. This is true agoraphobia. With help, however, extreme agoraphobics can learn to overcome their fear. The first step is usually medication to block the panic attacks. Then the really hard work starts. A program of gradual, controlled re-exposure to the feared places and situations must be undertaken. It takes a great deal of courage and commitment on the part of the patient. The therapist should be experienced in dealing with panic disorders. For patients who are afraid to leave home unattended, therapy could begin by spending a few minutes a day on the front porch. As confidence is gained, they move out first to the sidewalk, and then to the driveway, then they take short strolls. Relaxation exercises, biofeedback, and self-hypnosis are some of the tools used to cope with the anxiety that comes along the way. The whole process can take weeks or months, and the treatment usually depends on the frequency and extent of previous panic attacks.

As I have mentioned, the longer the panic attacks have been allowed to persist, the more difficult they are to manage. But when managed carefully with a combination of medication and behavioral therapy, there is a very high incidence of success. We would like ultimately to be able to predict which prolapse patients are likely to have panic disorder, and prevent it entirely. It would be helpful to monitor patients with high potential for panic attacks for signs of stress and potential triggers and, perhaps, to initiate preventive treatment. Many studies suggest that the tendency to develop panic attacks does run in families. Other studies have indicated that a history of school phobia is usually common in people who develop panic disorder as adults. These further support our contention that some people have a biologically inherited sensitive nervous system from birth. It will take years of careful study and follow-up to determine whether early detection efforts are going to have lasting benefits. But the combination of proper therapy and motivation results in a very high success rate, and I have seen panic disorder patients return to a thoroughly enjoyable life.

9 Putting It All Together — A Comprehensive Approach to Living with MVP

I hope this text has given you some of the information you need to take control of your life and of the uncomfortable and frightening symptoms of MVP. I also hope that I have conveyed the idea that there is no such thing as magic when you are seeking good health. No short cuts are allowed.

Each component of this program is important. As Figure 9-1 suggests, each element, exercise, dietary modifications, fluid intake, medications, and above all positive mental attitude, is essential to assure success.

I cannot choose one component of the program that is more important than the others. Any single component alone cannot control the problem. Dietary modifications are essential to the balance of the autonomic nervous system. Adequate fluid intake assures normal blood pressure and controls some of the uncomfortable symptoms that can be experienced with MVP. The importance of exercise can not be underestimated. Without a positive mental attitude, however, I doubt that anyone can muster the emotional energy to begin, much less stick with this or any program.

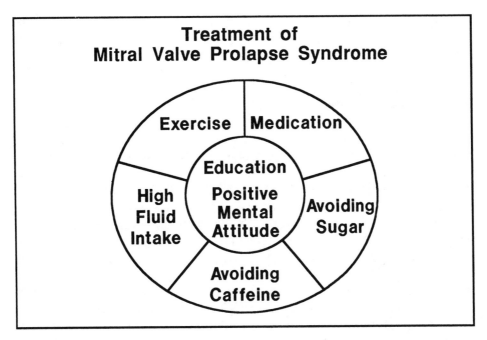

Figure 9-1

Start today! Don't put it off. Realize that you are the captain of your own ship and the master of your own fate, that you can no longer blame others for stress, or even rotten luck for your condition. Take control of and responsibility for your own health and happiness. Just as no other individual can make you happy, no other individual can make you healthy. You must do this for yourself. The first step in this process is often the realization that you can indeed make changes in your life and that you can succeed in this program. You need not feel helpless and out of control for another day. If you follow the self-help steps outlined in this book and still are not feeling as well as you think you should, there is additional help available (from psychologist or a physician), but remember that most of the plan needs to be implemented by you.

Be Nice To Yourself

This next recommendation may sound like it contradicts what I've been saying throughout the book. You must be nice to yourself and pay attention to others. Let me explain. Be nice to yourself by treating yourself to whatever you can afford in the way of luxuries—but not sweets or other dietary no-no's. They need not be expensive — a good book, a walk in the park, a soothing shower, or a healthful dinner out. If you have a few dollars to spare, try a manicure, or better yet a pedicure, a massage, a good movie (a comedy) or a lovely dinner by candlelight (skip the wine). All of these activities say "I'm special, and I'm worth the time and effort it takes to make me feel and look good."

By being nice to others I mean that you should do good deeds for others occasionally. Most prominent philosophers advise that the quickest way to get over the blues and depression is to do something for someone else in need. When you have been feeling poorly for a long time, you often have to act as though you feel well in order to begin to feel better. Look around to find out what you can do for others. Those of us in the medical profession need not look very far to find many people less fortunate than ourselves, such as the physically handicapped, the mentally impaired, or the homeless. Do something nice for someone else. Visit a nursing home or a hospital. Work with an activity in your church. Donate one evening a week to a local soup kitchen, or drive an elderly neighbor to the store. Perhaps a member of your family would enjoy a special evening out. Any number of activities that mean a great deal to the recipient will make you feel great. Are you starting to get the idea? I hope you will see that it is now time to begin to focus on something other than your own body. You may have been feeling poorly perhaps for a long time, but it is now time to put that behind you. Turn your attention to those activities and ideas outside yourself that will begin to bring you back into the mainstream of life. Not only will you feel better about yourself, but others will notice the difference in you immediately. Remember that those individuals who constantly talk about their loneliness, depression, illness, or the like are not very much fun to be with. Even those who love you the most will get tired eventually of hearing nothing but complaining about health problems. Develop an interest, and you will be interesting. Almost invariably, if you have a new interest, someone will be interested in hearing about it. Stop being bored with life, and your life will not be boring. Always remember to accentuate the positive side of life. The old adage that some individuals see a cup as half empty and others half full is a great example. All of us have half empty days when we see the world a little negatively. But try to limit those days. The optimist is a much happier individual than the pessimist. By taking control of your life and taking responsibility for your health, wellness, and happiness you can fill your life with joy and fulfillment. Good Luck!

10 Twenty Most Frequently Asked Questions About MVP

Q: *If I was born with it, why did I not have problems until I was 20 years old?*

A: Most patients report that some event preceded the onset of symptoms. The event can be either physical or psychological. The body perceives all stressors as biochemical insults. We believe that the biochemical event associated with the stress stimulates the imbalance in the autonomic nervous system. This imbalance, or "roller coaster" pattern, can continue until the body is returned to chemical balance.

Q: *I have two daughters. Should I have them checked for MVP?*

A: MVP is a physical variation that one or both of your daughters may have inherited from you. Remember that most people with MVP never have symptoms. I don't believe that it would be wise to introduce a mind-set for a medical problem that may never happen in an impressionable youngster who is just developing her body image. I think the best way to handle this is to teach your children through your example the importance of healthful habits for daily nutrition and exercise. You might also mention your concern to your pediatrician. If he hears the clicking sound with his stethoscope, he may recommend antibiotics prior to dental work, for example. I would handle this matter-of-factly and not produce needless anxiety.

Q: *Why do I need antibiotics before dental procedures?*

A: When dental procedures are performed, bacteria are released into the blood that can (very rarely) lodge on the mitral valve, producing an infection known as endocarditis. These infections though rare may be quite serious. As I mention in the text, many physicians do *not* recommend antibiotics. They believe that the chances of an infection are so remote that there is greater risk of a reaction to antibiotics. This argument has some merit, particularly with individuals who have a number of allergies to drugs. In individuals without allergies, however, I believe that it is prudent to take the antibiotics to be as safe as possible. I have included in Chapter 6 the most recent recommendations for antibiotics for dental procedures. As always you should ask your doctor's opinion; he or she should also know if these recommendations have been revised.

Q: *Can dysautonomia impair the sex drive?*

A: Yes. The autonomic nervous system is very important in the sexual function of the body, for both arousal and orgasm. When the autonomic nervous system is out of balance, some difficulty can result. It should be noted, however, that this is quite uncommon. I believe that most of the sexual difficulties I have found in my patients are due to fatigue and fear of symptoms during intercourse. These problems should be discussed frankly with your doctor or your psychologist, because they can result in marital problems.

Q: *Will I need to have a heart valve replacement?*

A: In my experience, probably not. Some individuals with severe valvular problems require replacement in time. But I don't believe that this is the case for routine MVP. In most cases, the heart functions well and a valve replacement is not needed. Further, it should be emphasized for very desperate and symptomatic individuals that dysautonomia — which is the source of symptoms in MVP — is not improved by valve replacement. After valve replacement an individual must be on blood thinners, *anticoagulants*, for the rest of his or her life. This is not without risk. Strokes and hemorrhage following valve replacement are not uncommon.

Q: *For years I have been told that my problems are "just nerves," I'm so discouraged. How much of these problems are really due to nerves?*

A: All of it! Not the psychological problems type of "nerves" that we generally mean but rather the autonomic nervous system. Remember that a variation in shape of a heart valve couldn't possibly have much to do with irritable bowel syndrome or migraine headaches. The autonomic nervous system is the culprit. This does not mean, however, that the individual with MVP is an emotionally unstable individual.

Q: *I snow-ski. When I go to high altitudes my heart goes crazy. What can I do? Is it safe to ski with MVP?*

A: By all means continue skiing. It is one of the most pleasurable of all activities. All of us have rapid heart rates when we go to high elevations. Individuals with MVP are much more aware of theirs, and their heart rate may be somewhat more elevated than the average. Several things will help. First, be in good physical condition when you go to high altitudes. Try to arrive by mid day, and then relax — don't try to ski that afternoon. Eat a light dinner, and try to rest. You may find it difficult to sleep, but rest. The next day take it very easy, and quit early. By the third day you should be fine. It also helps considerably to force fluids during your trip. Ski destinations are almost always quite dry, and the central heating and fireplaces tend to dry the air further, increasing the chance for dehydration and worsening of your symptoms. Start pushing fluids before you board the airplane, and continue to do so for several days. Also make sure before you go that you are not anemic. Many females are, and this can dramatically worsen the altitude effects.

Q: *I seem to have problems with air travel. Can anything help?*

A: This depends on whether your problems are the worsening symptoms that accompany the dehydration of jet travel or panic attacks that are common on airplanes. If your problems are increased tachycardia and mild shortness of breath, forcing fluids could help. Once again, remember, no caffeine or sugar. If the problem tends to be panic, the solution is a bit more complicated. As with all dysautonomia, the panic attacks tend to clear when everything is brought back into balance. The human being is a creature of habit and constantly tries to defend himself against unpleasant experiences. If you have a history of panic attacks when you get on an airplane, you may need more than the usual amount of help because you have learned to expect this reaction. Medications and a good psychologist should be able to overcome these problems. Travel is one of life's great pleasures and should not be avoided.

Q: *Can I get disability insurance payments for my MVP?*

A: Absolutely not! I have been working with MVP patients for a number of years and I have never seen anyone succeed in an attempt to collect disability benefits due to this condition, nor would I encourage such a pursuit. Some MVP patients are incapacitated due to psychiatric problems, but not because of MVP. With the tremendous number of individuals who have MVP, it would literally bankrupt the nation's economy if such a precedent were set. There is other help available!

Q: *How many individuals in our country have MVP?*

A: Millions. Most have no idea that they have this variation. It is estimated that between 10 and 20 percent of the population has it. In doing research on MVP, one of the more difficult tasks is to find individuals without MVP to use for comparison.

Q: *Can MVP be cured?*

A: MVP is an anatomical variation that is inherited. You were born with that variation, and it does not change. The symptoms that can accompany MVP can be controlled by lifestyle modifications and sometimes medication.

Q: *Why do more women than men have MVP?*

A: I'm not absolutely certain that more women do have MVP than men. I see many male patients. In fact one fourth of my MVP patients are men. It is known that women seek medical care much more readily than men. It is also culturally much more acceptable for women to complain of rather vague symptoms than it is for men. As I have mentioned, MVP symptoms, particularly panic, can be almost emasculating to a man. When men do seek care, it is usually for chest pain that they assume is heart disease.

Q: *Can I donate blood?*

A: Because the MVP patient is sensitive to changes in blood volume, donating blood can sometimes precipitate symptoms, just as dehydration from flulike illnesses and air travel can. There is no absolute contraindication to donating blood but caution should be exercised. If you are an individual with a tendency to low blood pressure, you are likely to have more symptoms after donating. If this has never been a problem, you probably will do well if you force fluids and have a very light snack prior to donation, and be sure to force fluids following donation.

Q: *Can I safely become pregnant?*

A: Yes. If you are anticipating pregnancy, be sure to check with your doctor first about discontinuing medication. I recommend that all medications be discontinued during pregnancy. The good news is that with the increasing blood volume during pregnancy, symptoms often disappear. Following delivery, with the fatigue that comes from late hours and to drop in blood volume, symptoms can recur. Care should be taken to assure a good diet and adequate fluid intake.

Q: *My symptoms seem to be worse when I drink alcoholic beverages. Can I safely drink occasionally?*

A: Once again, there is no absolute contraindication to an occasional drink. Alcohol, remember, is loaded with yeast, which is probably the most common allergen. It also tends to promote dehydration. Some forms of alcohol seem to be worse than others. As with everything else, moderation is the key. If you are like many MVP patients, you may find that the way you feel after only one or two drinks makes drinking not worth the price you have to pay.

Q: *What medications, other than the cardiac medications, should I avoid?*

A: I have included in Chapter 6 a listing of drugs that can be purchased over the counter and that contain substances that are frequently a problem for MVP patients. This list is by no means complete. You should check with your pharmacist or physician if you have a tendency to be very sensitive to medications, and above all, always read labels.

Q: *I have recently read an article in a medical journal that I didn't understand very well, but one item got my attention. It said that MVP was associated with sudden death. I'm terrified. Is this true?*

A: I read the same article. This is surely a very scary thing for a patient with MVP to hear, particularly if he or she suffers from chest pain and shortness of breath. The patient may think that every attack represents "the big one." Let me make every effort to reassure you why I and many others believe that this simply is not the case. I probably have seen about as many prolapse patients as anyone; I have a patient file of more than 3,000 patients. I have never lost a single patient to sudden death. My colleagues, and I have many, can contribute several thousand more cases, and they have never seen a case of sudden death in an MVP patient without other problems. Most often, sudden death occurs in an individual with disease of the coronary arteries. As previously mentioned, that is entirely different from MVP. Older individuals with MVP may also have coronary disease and thus may be susceptible to sudden death. Remember that MVP occurs in up to 20 percent of the population. If a study demonstrated that more than 20 percent of the cases of sudden death had MVP and no other problem, I might be worried. I have never seen a study that has demonstrated that. Another cause of sudden death is a problem in the electrical system of the heart. It is not known to be associated with MVP, and it is extremely rare. I hope you find this reassuring.

Q: *My most disturbing symptom is a "lump in my throat" that makes it difficult to swallow. What causes this?*

A: I honestly don't know. Several of my patients have told me this. I believe that it must be musculo-skeletal in origin — that is, tightness of the muscles of the chest and throat. In my experience it almost always goes away when the system is returned to balance.

Q: *Why are my hands and feet as cold as ice?*

A: The autonomic nervous system controls the contraction and relaxation of the blood vessels of the hands and feet as well as the rest of the body. Often if the autonomic nervous system is out of balance, too much constriction of these vessels results and thus cold hands and feet. Some individuals report that the tips of their fingers can become blue due to lack of circulation. This is known as Raynaud's phenomenon. MVP is one of the common causes of this.

Q: *Why am I so tired all of the time?*

A: Fatigue is the most commonly reported symptom of MVP. There are a number of reasons this occurs. Once again, the imbalance in the autonomic nervous system tends to result in the abnormal constriction or relaxation of the blood vessels and can somewhat limit the blood supply to the large muscles, resulting in the build up of chemicals known as lactic acid. Lactic acid produces fatigue. The other very common source of fatigue is the tendency to be very much out of shape, or deconditioned. The less we do, the less we feel like doing. When symptoms occur and result in fatigue or more symptoms, the individual tends to do less and less. The old adage of "what you don't use, you lose" applies here. Our muscles need activity to remain strong. A vicious cycle of fatigue must be broken by gently returning to physical activities and consistently striving to achieve a state of optimal conditioning.

Glossary

ANS — See *autonomic nervous system.*

ANST — See *autonomic nervous system testing.*

Anxiety attack — Sudden unexplained feelings of fear and dread often accompanied by intense discomfort and the need to flee; may or may not be accompanied by rapid heartbeat and shortness of breath.

Atrium — One of two upper chambers of the heart.

Autonomic nervous system — The involuntary nervous system composed of two parts — sympathetic and parasympathetic; innervates every system in the body and controls heart rate, respiration rate, digestion, and sleep, as well as many other functions.

Autonomic nervous system testing — A series of tests designed to measure the responses of the autonomic nervous system for the purpose of choosing medication to relieve unpleasant symptoms that result from an imbalance in this system.

Beta blockers — A class of drugs (Inderal, Tenormin, and Clonidine are examples) that may be used to relieve certain symptoms associated with mitral valve prolapse. Generally, this class of drugs slows the heart rate and decreases blood pressure.

Calcium channel blocker — A class of drugs (Cardizem and Nifedipine are examples) that may be used to relieve certain symptoms of mitral valve prolapse. As a general rule these drugs are used to control chest pain and elevated blood pressure.

Cardiac — Having to do with the heart.

Cardiologist — A medical doctor who has had additional training to qualify him or her to treat and diagnose diseases of the heart and blood vessels.

Cholesterol — A fatlike substance that is in many foods; tends to collect in the walls of blood vessels and leads to atherosclerosis, coronary artery disease that predisposes to heart attack.

Conditioning — Exercise which is of sufficient frequency and intensity to result in improvement of cardiovascular and respiratory fitness.

Deconditioning — The state the results from prolonged inactivity and results in decreased functional capacity, unstable blood pressure, and inappropriate heart rate responses to minimal activity. It also results in undue amounts of fatigue with only small amounts of activity.

Dysautonomia — An imbalance in the autonomic nervous system that results in symptoms such as rapid heartbeat, fatigue, chest pain, shortness of breath, and sometimes panic and anxiety attacks.

Echocardiogram — A diagnostic test that utilizes sound waves to visualize heart structures. The test is painless and is the one most often used to determine the presence of mitral valve prolapse.

Endocarditis — Infection of the innermost layer of the heart.

Family medicine specialist — A physician who is specifically trained in the treatment of general medical problems in patients of all ages; formerly referred to as general practitioner.

Fibrocystic breast disease — Benign (noncancerous) condition associated with lumpy, painful breasts in women.

Internist — A physician who has received special training in the diagnosis and treatment of internal medical problems of all kinds in adult men and women.

Irritable bowel — Tendency for diarrhea, constipation, or both; may be worsened by stressful situations and may be accompanied by abdominal pain.

Metabolic stress test — Exercise test utilizing a special piece of equipment that measures the oxygen consumption of the body (how efficiently the muscles of the body use oxygen), generally considered the "gold standard" of fitness.

Mitral valve — The structure that separates the upper chamber from the lower chamber on the left side of the heart.

Mitral valve prolapse (MVP) — Billowing upward of the mitral valve into the upper chamber of the heart; often associated with chest pain, shortness of breath, tachycardia, and other symptoms.

Migraine headache — Severe headache, often on one side of the head, that may be preceded by visual sensations or accompanied by nausea.

MVP — See mitral valve prolapse.

Neurologist — A physician specializing in the diagnosis and treatment of diseases of the brain and nerves.

Palpitations — Sensations of "skipping" or "flip-flop" of the heartbeat. Rapid or normal rate may be accompanied by a pause following a particularly strong beat.

Panic attack — Sudden, intense, unexplained sensation of dread and fear accompanied by intense urge to flee, may be precipitated by some external event such as flying, or may occur spontaneously; may be accompanied by rapid heart beat and or shortness of breath.

Prognosis — Prediction of the outcome of a situation; that is, a good prognosis predicts a favorable outcome.

Psychiatrist — A physician specializing in the diagnosis and treatment of emotional disorders.

Psychologist — An individual trained to administer and interpret psychological tests and specialized in psychotherapy and counseling.

Syncope — Fainting.

Syndrome — A group of symptoms associated with the same condition.

Tachycardia — Rapid heartbeat.

Temporo-Mandibular Joint Disease (TMJ) — Malalignment of the jaw that results in headaches and other symptoms. May be associated with mitral valve prolapse.

Ventricle — Lower chamber of the heart.

Suggested Reading

Seagrave, Ann. *Free from Fears*. Poseidon Press, New York, 1987.

James, Muriel. *Born to Win*. Signet Books, New York, 1978.

Shaevitz, Marjorie. *The Superwoman Syndrome*. Warner Books, New York, 1984.

Handly, Robert. *Anxiety and Panic Attacks; Their Cause and Cure*. Fawcett Crest, New York, 1985.

Dyer, Wayne, M.D. *Your Erroneous Zones*. Avon Books, New York, 1976.

Cushner, Harold S. *When Bad Things Happen to Good People*. Avon Books, New York, 1983.

Brody, Jane. *Jane Brody's Nutrition Book*. Bantam Books, New York, 1982.

Dufty, William. *Sugar Blues*. Warner Books, New York, 1975.

Cooper, Mildred and Kenneth. *Aerobics for Women*. Bantam Books, New York, 1972.

Alberti, Robert. *Stand-up, Speak-out*. Pocket Books, New York, 1970.

Kuntzleman, Charles. *The Complete Book of Walking*. Pocket Books of New York, New York, 1979.

Morris, Ronald. *PMS Prove Program on How to Recognize and Treat PMS*. Berkley Books, New York, 1983.

Weller, Charles. *How to Live with Hypoglycemia*. Jove Books, New York, 1968.

Sheehan, David. *The Anxiety Disease*. Bantam Books, New York, 1983.

Greene, Melvin. *Living Fear Free*. Warner Books, New York, 1985.

Newman, Fredric. *Fighting Fear — The Eight Week Program for Treating Your Own Phobias*. Bantam Books, New York, 1985.

Meyers, Casey. *Aerobic Walking*. Vintage Books, New York, 1987.

Yanker, Gary. *The Complete Book of Exercise and Walking*. Contemporary Books of Chicago, Chicago, 1983.

Marchetti, Albert, M.D. *Walking Book.* Scarbrough Books, New York, 1980.

John Pleas, PhD. *Walking.* W. W. Norton Co., New York, 1981.

Cooper, Kenneth, M.D. *The Aerobics Program for Total Well Being.* Bantam Books, New York, 1982.

Colvert, Bailey. *Fit or Fat.* Houghton Mifflin Co., Boston, 1977.

Benson, Herbert. *The Relaxation Response.* Avon Books, New York, 1975.

Kuntzleman, Charles. *The Complete Book of Walking.* Pocket Books of New York, New York, 1979.

Cannon, Geoffrey. *Dieting Makes You Fat.* Pocket Books of New York, New York, 1983.

Davis, Francyne. *The Low Blood Sugar Cookbook.* Bantam Books, New York, 1973.

Spodnik, Jean. *The 35 Plus Diet for Women.* Harper and Row, New York, 1987.

Steincrohn, Peter. *Low Blood Sugar.* Signet Books New York, New York, 1972.

Weeks, Claire. *Peace from Nervous Suffering.* Bantam Books, New York, 1972.

Bailey, Colvert. *Fit or Fat Target Diet.* Houghton Miffin Co., 1984.

Ardell, Donald B. *High-Level Wellness.* Ten Speed Press, 1977.

Index

About the Author

Lyn Frederickson holds a Master of Science in Cardiovascular Nursing from the University of Alabama at Birmingham. She has extensive experience in the care of critically ill cardiac patients and in cardiovascular rehabilitation. Mrs. Frederickson directs and was instrumental in the establishment of the Mitral Valve Prolapse Center of Alabama, located at Baptist Medical Center Montclair, Birmingham, Alabama. The Center is the first facility of its kind in the world, specializing in the diagnosis, treatment, and rehabilitation of patients with mitral valve prolapse syndrome. Patients with mitral valve prolapse syndrome are referred to Mrs. Frederickson from all over the world. She has authored numerous articles, books, video tapes, and materials for patient and family education regarding cardiovascular diseases. Mrs. Frederickson may be contacted at P.O. Box 20148, Birmingham, AL 35216.

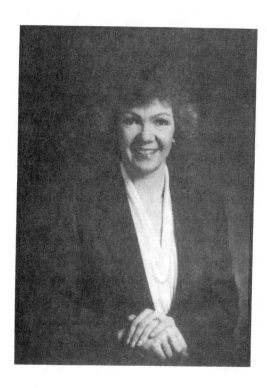

mvprolapse.com
mitral.com
medexpert.net

Kevin Thomas, MD.
       St Joe's
   Dysautonomia

Lifewaves.
Heartwaves
       Irving
   Dr. Dardick
   Dr. Goldberger

Johns Hopkins - muscle group
            treating girl